GREAT SEX NEVER GETS OLD

Health, Hormones, and Having it All After Forty

KIMBERLY CUNNINGHAM

CUNNINGHAM CLINIC
DENVER, CO

Praise for
Great Sex Never Gets Old

"Cunningham Clinic is by far the best aesthetics/HRT provider I have EVER experienced! Kimberly, the owner, is the most knowledgeable medical provider I've ever worked with in this space! She cares, she constantly increases her knowledge base, which is already huge, and she hires only the best of the best. I've seen Kimberly for years, and I also go to other staff for many services. If an aesthetician/medical professional is employed by Cunningham Clinic, rest assured they possess the highest level of skill/expertise and are every bit as lovely as a person as Kimberly. This clinic is truly such a gift to me, and I strongly recommend them."

"Kimberly is AMAZING! Patient, kind, a great listener, extremely helpful information and proactive rather than reactive in her recommendations. I will tell many folks about her because she is a truly caring and smart practitioner. I was deeply impressed!"

"I've been going to Cunningham Clinic for years, they are amazing. I went in today to have blood drawn for the Biote® program. They took my blood and for the first time ever, it didn't hurt! I highly recommend them. They are very knowledgeable and gentle. I'm so happy with all of their services!"

"Consummate professionals who care about their clients. I have worked with them on Biote® and it has made a big difference in my energy level. My M.D. was also impressed with what we accomplished with the combination of the pellet and the supplements when I had other health issues."

"Kimberly is professional, fast, knows her stuff, and is a wonderful teacher. She helped me through a health issue that required extra research and time with no problems or extra charges. Always a terrific experience at Cunningham Clinic!"

"I have done Biote® for two years, and I was looking for help with Biote® in the Denver area. I had my first appointment with Kimberly this week. I was so impressed with how well she listened and truly loves helping people feel better. I learned a lot and felt very cared for. Kimberly is very thorough, and I did not feel like she was in a hurry. Excited to find the Cunningham Clinic."

"I have struggled with hormone replacement for quite some time. Some people I have seen didn't seem to care about consistency or my symptoms. Kimberly is not only intelligent, but she's also very consistent. I'm thrilled to have found her and look forward to this health journey together. Highly recommend."

"Kimberly is a true artist in both aesthetics and balancing out hormones. Without reservation, I am recommending her to friends. It is so refreshing to be her patient; she absolutely puts my needs and desires as strict guiding principles. The results I have achieved have been incredible. I cannot thank her enough."

Copyright © 2023 by Kimberly Cunningham.

All rights reserved. No part of this book may be reproduced in any written, electronic, recording, or photocopying without written permission of the publisher or author. The exception would be in the case of brief quotations embodied in articles or reviews and pages where permission is specifically granted by the publisher or author.

Cunningham Clinic/ Great Sex Never Gets Old

Printed in the United States of America

Although every precaution has been taken to verify the accuracy of the information contained herein, the author and publisher assume no responsibility for any errors or omissions. No liability is assumed for damages that may result from the use of information contained within.

Great Sex Never Gets Old/ Kimberly Cunningham -- 2nd ed.

ISBN 978-8-9881143-0-7 Print Edition

LCCN Number: 2023906165

CONTENTS

Introduction vii
It Ain't Over 'til It's Over 1
Wellness Check 7
Women and Menopause 19
Hormone Replacement Therapy for Women 31
Men and Middle Age 41
Other Hormones Matter 51
Getting Hormones Into the Body 61
Side Effects 77
A Year in the Life 89
The Hormones Are Fixed, But 95
Treating Erectile Dysfunction 111
Sexy Time 121
Attachment 133
Let's Do It! 143
References 149
About the Author 175
HRT Checklist For Women and Men 177

INTRODUCTION

Not too many years ago, I went to my primary care provider with a list of complaints: "I've gained weight, I can't sleep, and I don't feel well."

"Welcome to your forties," he said.

As in, welcome to the next half of your life where you have no choice but to accept feeling fat, tired, and unhappy?

"Do you actually tell people this all day long?" I asked.

As a busy, physically active former emergency room nurse practitioner who'd worked in geriatrics and internal medicine practices, I knew that age brings on physiological changes for both men and women. I also knew there had to be a better way than just telling clients to give up and simply learn to accept the inevitable.

And then, halfway through my second pregnancy, my pelvis broke. It just broke! Over a period of ten days, I went from a person who walked to a person who shuffled to a person who couldn't move without extreme pain. It felt like my pelvis was splitting apart with every step. As it turned out, my pelvis actually was splitting apart. The surgeons called it *spontaneous pelvic integrity failure in pregnancy*, and it is so rare, none of them had ever seen it before. But it happened to me—and I still had a baby to grow.

INTRODUCTION

The next 14 weeks were a terrifying stretch of seconds, each one seeming to last a year. Through the work of an incredible team, one of whom even drove across town to do in-home visits for me, they dragged me through just enough days to give birth to a healthy baby boy.

This once-in-a-million happenstance was due to a combination of Ehlers-Danlos syndrome and a congenitally misshapen pelvis. Ehlers-Danlos is a genetic defect that causes connective tissue to be hypermobile. If connective tissue is thought of like a knit sweater, most people are born with a tight weave. People with Ehlers-Danlos are born with more of an "open weave" which can lead to a high fracture load, joints that are easily dislocated and, in *win the lottery and get struck by lightning on the same day* odds, pelvic integrity failure in pregnancy. I didn't know I had this defect, so there wasn't a way to avoid my injury, but my life, literally fell apart.

Before my pregnancy, I was a fitness enthusiast and had even finished in the top ten at a sprint triathlon. Following the delivery of my son, I endured more than ten surgeries, including multiple rounds of hardware in, hardware out, and repeated attempts to fuse my broken pelvis, which left me only able to shuffle around, and no further than 500 steps a day. I had to use a scooter in stores like Target, and I needed a wheelchair to get through the airport.

As for sex with a broken pelvis, it was a non-starter.

For the next four years, I tried everything I could think of to get out of my wheelchair—I did ten hours a week of physical therapy, often working so hard I would vomit mid-workout. I ate like I was training for a race, cutting all inflammatory foods, and consuming 120 grams of protein per day. I endured as much pain as I could handle, assuming I would gain my strength and health back. The problem was, even with the advice of 15 specialists, I simply wasn't recovering.

During that time, my former employer (a large HMO) asked me to come back. I was so weak and exhausted, all I could consider was a six-hour urgent care shift once a week, only in the smallest location utilizing my cane for short distances, and then rest all week to do it again.

In trying to stitch together a semblance of a life and get back to work again, I signed up for a day-long continuing medical education lab review class. Seeing as I hadn't read a lab result in four years, the class—which focused on the fundamentals of bloodwork—seemed like it might even be interesting.

As I entered the 200-seat lecture hall, a colorful patchwork shoulder bag caught my eye up near the front. I decided to take the empty seat beside its owner thinking a woman who owned such a lively bag might be fun to get to know. As I labored up the steps toward the open seat and the handbag, I realized I knew the woman. In fact, we'd gone to nursing school together at the University of Colorado.

Needless to say, she was extremely curious about the visible changes to my health and asked what had happened. During the breaks, I filled her in about the challenges I'd faced and how I was still having so many problems—including exhaustion and the inability to regain any strength or muscle mass.

"Have you tried Biote®?" she asked.

"Biote®?" I responded, wondering what it was and how I'd never heard of it.

She proceeded to give me a crash course in American versus European hormone replacement, testosterone replacement for men AND women, and Biote® pellet therapy. Her description not only made sense medically but resonated with what I'd been feeling health-wise.

This "chance" meeting set me on the path to an entirely different way of approaching endocrinology and healthy aging that not only changed my life but enabled me to help many others. As a science nerd, I researched every study I could find, nationally and internationally. What wasn't taught in the United States at the time, but is now becoming accepted as common practice, is that when a woman's testosterone falls below 30, she likely cannot grow muscle. Below 20, most women cannot grow bone. I had my own blood tested and learned my testosterone level was at *seven,* which explained why I kept working harder at getting fit but was only breaking my body down with no possibility of building it back up. I realized I had spent years in a literal nosedive, getting weaker, sicker, and fatter at an accelerated pace.

The Biote® method is a way of getting hormones back into humans – testosterone for men and testosterone with or without estrogen for women—via slow-release, dissolvable pellets implanted in the subcutaneous fat in the hip or the flank.

Within three weeks of my first round of pellets, I was sleeping through the night. During that third week, I also woke up and realized the pain I'd been living with—like sharp teeth constantly biting into me day and night was gone. I stopped being a human barometer, reacting with internal discomfort to weather changes. I was able to stop the pain medicine I'd been taking for years. Six weeks later, my muscle tone started coming back. Soon, I was out of the wheelchair for good.

Incredibly, my sex drive, which had been entirely nonexistent from being in constant pain, partially wheelchair bound, and devoid of testosterone, came roaring back.

Six months later, and feeling healthy and happy, I rented a small space in the back of a local med spa in Denver to open a small practice helping other people who were suffering like I had been. A lot of my first clients were friends, mostly female, who'd had a front row seat to my transition from triathlete to wheelchair bound and then back to great health.

"Whatever it is you're doing, sign me up," they said.

The results were startling and measurable for my clients as well. Referrals began to pour in from my first clients' friends, extended family members, and miracle of miracles, husbands who had some balancing needs of their own.

By the end of the first year, I had 100 clients. Now, at Cunningham Clinic, we have in excess of 1200. I've had to invest in multiple lab coats because of the near daily make-up stains on my right shoulder from the "ugly crying" of women (and men) whose test results proved they weren't making up the symptoms that had had them feeling off-kilter for years.

Years later, it's still the best feeling in the world to help people enhance their health, lives, and yes, their sex lives.

IT AIN'T OVER 'TIL IT'S OVER

It's the end of the day, and you're in bed, exhausted. You want something—a cookie, to have sex with your partner, or maybe watch TV—but definitely not all three, and you really don't care which.

Sound a little too familiar?

People come into my office every day complaining they're just holding on by their fingernails. Whether it's working, parenting, socializing, working out, or traveling, they never feel *un*-tired. They are typically in possession of what I call a supplement graveyard—as in every Facebook, YouTube, try this, and use that product promising to increase energy. They've dabbled in Keto, Paleo, and have definitely tried to cut "the enemy" aka carbs from their diets. As for increasing stamina, the list is endless: protein shakes, B-12 shots, energy drinks . . .

The truth is symptoms of what my husband likes to call "olditis" begin to creep in for women and men at around age 35. There is fatigue, weight gain, loss of muscle tone, and diminished libido. They feel like they can get the machine to work, but it's a Herculean effort to get started and keep it going. At around age 50, the underlying sense of malaise and weight gain is then joined by a host of annoying and often debilitating symptoms. For women, there are the hot flashes that start in the chest, explode up through the head, and leave them feeling gross, sweaty, and needing a shower. Night sweats, hair loss, mood changes, vaginal dryness, and tissue integrity changes in the vaginal vault add to the pain and misery. For men, there is increasing erectile dysfunction so prevalent it has spawned a multi-billion dollar male enhancement product industry.

Why? For women, perimenopause and menopause—the cessation or the stopping of ovulation—is responsible for the general umbrella of symptoms. It's called andropause in men when the testosterone falls so low, he loses sexual performance and other functions. Decreased hormones are behind a lot of the dysfunction, and teasing out which hormone is causing what issue is key to getting his body and sex life back.

Decreased estrogen levels result in hot flashes, weight gain, and dryness in the vagina. Sex becomes painful and there doesn't seem to be enough lubrication to rectify the problem. Like men, women also lose testosterone as they age. Without enough testosterone, fatigue and night sweats increase, and libido drops right off. Worse, as testosterone falls, the risk for the conditions and diseases of inflammation—cancer, arthritis, diabetes, high blood pressure—all go up.

As they say, getting old isn't for the faint of heart, but I'm here to tell you it doesn't have to be! By fixing the imbalances in thyroid, Vitamin B_{12} and D levels, testosterone, and estrogen (in women when necessary) just about everybody can turn back their internal clock, feel, look like and be a 30-year-old version of themselves.

In this book we will talk about how great sex never gets old. In order to do so, however, we need to talk about the hormonal and physiological changes that happen before and around menopause and, what is sometimes jokingly referred to as *manopause*. There are a lot of factors that go into sexual wellness. Like with high blood pressure or diabetes, you have to have your treatment algorithm, so we're going to talk about preventative care that is actually preventative. We're going to talk about hormone replacement therapy. We're going to talk about getting balanced, which leads to better sleep, better sex, better relationships, and less depression. We're going to talk about medical interventions that may be necessary. And then, we're going to talk about shopping for toys and how to set the mood, plan for, and enjoy some really, really good sexy time.

Are you ready?

FACTS ABOUT MENOPAUSE

- 3500 women enter menopause daily in the United States.
- Symptoms of menopause may begin up to 15 years prior to menopause.
- Most women are affected in more ways than they realize.
- Most women do not ever "get over" or "get through" menopause completely even where they are completely asymptomatic.
- The average age of menopause is 51. Genetics, smoking, surgery, and ethnicity affect the age of menopause.
- The age your mom and sisters went through menopause should give you some clues about yourself.

In the years leading up to menopause, also known as perimenopause, women are likely to experience some or possibly all of these symptoms:

SYMPTOMS OF MENOPAUSE

- Irregular periods
- Vaginal dryness
- Hot flashes
- Chills
- Night sweats
- Sleep disturbances
- Mood changes
- Weight gain
- Slowed metabolism
- Thinning hair
- Dry skin
- Loss of breast fullness
- Loss of libido/sex drive

FACTS ABOUT ANDROPAUSE

As men age, testosterone levels and production of sperm gradually decrease. They experience physical and psychological symptoms as a result of these low levels. It is estimated that testosterone decreases about 10% every decade after men reach the age of 30. This decrease in testosterone and the development of symptoms is more gradual than what occurs in women. Approximately 30% of men in their 50s will experience symptoms of andropause caused by low testosterone levels. A person experiencing andropause may have a number of symptoms related to the condition and could be at risk of other serious health conditions such as osteoporosis without proper treatment.

SYMPTOMS OF ANDROPAUSE

- Low sex drive
- Fat redistribution, such as developing a large belly or "man boobs" (gynecomastia)
- Difficulty sleeping (insomnia) or increased tiredness
- Poor concentration and short-term memory
- Difficulties getting erections or erections that are not as strong as usual
- Lack of energy
- Depression
- Irritability and mood swings
- Loss of strength or muscle mass
- Reduced ability and desire to exercise
- Increased body fat
- Hot flashes
- Increased risk of cardiovascular problems
- Increased risk of osteoporosis

WELLNESS CHECK

At the Cunningham Clinic, 99% of our business is from referrals. New clients come in because they see a friend we've treated go from being cranky, tired, gaining weight, hair falling out and not interested in having sex to all of a sudden being vital, amorous again with their partner, having a smile on their face and full of energy.

We help everyone to achieve the same results by tailoring protocols to their specific health needs.

When a new client comes in, we do a complete medical history. For women, we need answers to specific questions: Do you still have a uterus? Are you in menopause or perimenopausal? What surgeries have you had? What medicines and supplements do you take? The list goes on, and is extensive, because we want as much information and as complete a picture as we can possibly get. For men, many of the same questions apply, but we also ask about erectile dysfunction—most have performance issues of one sort or another.

After we review the health history with the patient, we get the same labs that primary care doctors order including a CBC and a TSH. However, traditional general practitioners typically stop there and that's where our similarities end. We then order additional labs that provide detailed information about thyroid, Vitamin D and B$_{12}$, sugar metabolism, cholesterol levels and, of course, all of the sex hormones. These numbers tell a different, far more complete, health story.

**Do we age because we lose our hormones?
Or, do we lose our hormones because we age?**

HERE COME THE UGLY TEARS

One week after the labs are drawn, our clients come in for an hour-long meeting to go through exactly what their test results show.

In terms of thyroid, for example, the American Thyroid Society says you're "fine" if your TSH or thyroid stimulating hormone is between the range of 0.4 – 4 mIU / L. This reference range is often based on bloodwork analyzed by an amalgam of people who had blood drawn while they were hospitalized. In other words, the range considered normal is a mixture of everyone from an 18-year-old getting her appendix out to a 92 year-old in heart failure. How that's applicable or helpful to a 54 year-old woman with low energy, depression, and menopausal weight gain who's been told by multiple providers to *consider cutting calories,* I'm just not sure!

A lot of people have thyroids which make plenty of T4, but they're not converting it into the active form, which is free T3, and when they can't make that conversion anymore, it's called low Free T3 syndrome. As a result, their hair is falling out, they're gaining weight around their middle, they're cold all the time, and they can't think their way out of a box. It takes just a few more lines of lab work to tell the complete story of someone's thyroid and get them on the right path.

Vitamin D recommendations are also head scratchers. I've never understood why one of the biggest labs in the country devotes a full half inch of space to explaining that a Vitamin D level of 30-100 is within acceptable limits. Seeing as we've known for over 20 years that people with autoimmune diseases like allergies, asthma, and chronic pain need to be above 70 ng/ML to get their conditions under control, I have to wonder who is behind their insistence that this version of "normal" is optimal? For almost the last three years, we have had additional evidence-based data out of The University of Chicago Medicine showing that if your Vitamin D isn't above 60, your ability to fight COVID is greatly reduced as well.

While that lab believes it's important to explain that this broad Vitamin D range is acceptable, some of the other labs don't even give numbers, just whether the level is considered normal or abnormal with the reference range off to the side. In my opinion, industry standards like these are misleading at best. At worst, they can cause failures in proper endocrinologic treatment.

In my practice, we aren't treating clients to outdated or inappropriate reference ranges. For the best outcomes, we use an amalgam of functional medicine guidelines and European data sets. When I examine bloodwork from clients and compare the numbers to a healthy 30 year-old, an entirely different health picture emerges. Sometimes, the Vitamin D is terrible. At other times, the B12 is off. Most often, however, hormonal imbalances are responsible for the physical changes, sexual dysfunction, and inflammatory problems that bring people into Cunningham Clinic.

When someone comes in with depression, inability to focus, insomnia, asthma, allergies, or autoimmune conditions out of control, and I see their Vitamin D is at 19, we can fix that. If their blood work shows a loss of testosterone and/or estrogen, we get to work on the maladies we blame on getting older—everything from pelvic floor weakness and urinary incontinence to a total loss of sex drive.

"The bad news is it looks like Armageddon," I've been known to say to clients. "But the good news is I can fix it."

I always keep tissues in reach because, so often, there are tears. Not because people fear for their health, or are concerned about how I will go about getting their hormone levels balanced, but because they now know the symptoms they've been experiencing weren't in their head. They are relieved they're not crazy and they've finally found the health care provider who is going to, as I say, "Age you in reverse back as far as I can get you, and then hold you there for as long as I can."

When the happy, ugly crying starts, I am left with the makeup marks I have to launder out of the right shoulders of so many of my lab coats!

At that point, recommendations are made as to what is needed in terms of Vitamin D and/ or B_{12} supplements. We discuss thyroid medication, if necessary. Then we move on to what is usually the biggest issue of all: hormones.

THE ELEPHANT IN THE ROOM

Before going any further, we need to discuss the most common question asked of all healthcare providers in my field: Is hormone replacement therapy safe? We've all heard stories about perimenopausal hormone treatments causing cancer, and it's crucial to sort out the fear from the facts.

In 2003, part of the Women's Health Initiative study was stopped because of an uptick in breast cancer. In that study, research subjects were being treated for perimenopausal and menopausal symptoms with a synthetic oral estrogen derived from pregnant horses (whose foals are sent immediately to slaughter and then the mare is immediately reimpregnated, which I consider to be beyond deplorable) plus a synthetic progesterone called medroxyprogesterone.

In menopause, if a woman still has her uterus and she's getting estrogen, it needs to be opposed with progesterone or the uterine lining will grow too thick. This can cause bleeding and, eventually, an increased risk of uterine cancer.

In the Women's Health Initiative study, clients were either given Premarin (conjugated pregnant horse estrogen) if they didn't have a uterus, or Prempro, an oral combination of conjugated pregnant horse estrogen PLUS the synthetic medroxyprogesterone acetate if they still had their uterus. It turns out that the increased risk of breast cancer in that study was exclusive to the Prempro (estrogen plus synthetic progesterone) arm of the study. It was the synthetic progesterone arm of the study that may have showed the increased risk of breast growth and cancer, NOT the estrogen.

In the end, all but one of the researchers involved in the study recanted their claim that estrogen causes breast cancer. In fact, 20 years after that part of the Women's Health Initiative study ended, women who were in the Premarin (estrogen only) arm of the study are showing a *decrease* in the lifetime risk of breast cancer. Time will tell, but the data sets are starting to look like estrogen may even be breast protective in the absence of synthetic progesterone.

Most of us who practice HRT believe that if the original Women's Health Initiative study had prescribed micronized progesterone, which is a non-synthetic, bioidentical form of progesterone, the results would have shown that there was no increased risk of breast cancer. In other words, hormones that are molecularly identical to those found in humans do not show increased risk of breast or other cancers, and likely reduce the risk of solid tumor cancers, breast included.

Micronized progesterone (the one that is bioidentical) sounds like medroxyprogesterone (the synthetic version that may increase the risk of breast cancer), but it's a different covalent bond/molecular structure. The researchers and drug manufacturers used the wrong progesterone, put women at unnecessary risk, and erroneously frightened women away from much needed hormone replacement therapy.

During the decades while many U.S. women were scared away from hormone therapy and had few options to reduce their misery, researchers were engaged in a ten-year study of 1,000 women who were receiving bioidentical hormone replacement therapy. (Many of whom were BRCA1 and BRCA2 positive, which put them at greater risk for breast cancer.) In March 2021, the *European Journal of Breast Health* published a retrospective study which measured the breast cancer incidence in this group. They concluded that for those taking bioidentical estrogen, progesterone, and testosterone, there was actually a 38% reduction in the risk of breast cancer and a 59% reduction in the risk of invasive breast cancer. Not an increase, but a massive reduction in the risk of breast cancer.

The takeaways are many. Not only did the bioidentical study participants *not* develop breast cancer, but there was a huge reduction in the risk of breast cancer compared to women who did nothing. Seeing as breast cancer has been as high the number two killer of Americans over recent years, if we can reduce that by 38% in almost 60% of the population it's a massive shift in improved health outcomes.

Hormones change risk factors and improve outcomes on other fronts as well. In fact, the participants in the Women's Health Initiative study who were given estrogen and progesterone had better cardiovascular outcomes and better Alzheimer's outcomes than the women who didn't get any hormones—so even pregnant horse estrogen helps protect hearts and minds. If the women had gotten testosterone as well, they would have likely felt better, had a sex drive, not been sweaty at night, had greater bone density and muscle tone, and had some protection from carcinogens.

> ### *Dianne: Age 76*
> *It's amazing how many women my age don't do HRT because of that now debunked study back in the 2000s. I think a lot of women threw it over, never thought about it again, and just aged in place. However, a few of us are lucky enough to come across places like Cunningham Clinic.*
>
> *I've lost weight, my skin is firmer, and my neck no longer looks like a plucked chicken!*

A lot of people ask, "Can I have estrogen? There's a risk of breast cancer in my family."

The answer is almost always, yes. BRCA1 and BRCA2 are genetic changes that make a person more susceptible to the environmental impacts/damages that increase the risk of breast, ovarian and endometrial/uterine cancers. This means that person needs greater and more frequent surveillance in the form of mammography and pelvic ultrasound, not that they have to suffer through the second half of their life. I don't give women estrogen if they've had an estrogen-positive cancer in the past with a risk of recurrence, but they absolutely get testosterone for sex drive, muscle tone, and vascular engorgement. The whole functionality of the clitoris is testosterone-driven, and it's crucial for sexy time!

For women who can't take systemic estrogen but are far enough out from their estrogen-positive cancer treatment, they can certainly get transvaginal estrogen to plump up that vaginal vault. We can't help those women with the hot flashes, but we can get that vaginal vault integrity back and get them looking and feeling great.

FACTS ABOUT ESTROGEN

- Present in both men and women
- Large amounts in women, very small amounts in men
- Has OVER 400 functions in the body
    - ◊ Controls hot flashes
    - ◊ Maintains bone density in both women *and men*
    - ◊ Helps maintain memory
    - ◊ Maintains collagen in your skin
- Increases serotonin and dopamine the "happy" hormones in brain

I WANT WHAT SHE'S HAVING

In the years since I opened Cunningham Clinic, I've had the pleasure of seeing my clients thrive. I compare them to friends who, to the best of my knowledge, don't receive any kind of hormone replacement therapy. I treat my parents who love the way they look and feel. They have far fewer concerns about the aging process and lead more active and full lives than their friends who don't do hormone replacement therapy—all of whom are from a similar socioeconomic group, education level, and have the same access to healthcare. What they can do is different, what they can tolerate is different, and what they look like is different. It even shows in the comparative strength of their voices. Which is why when a person comes in and gets treated, the next thing you know, their entire family and friend group is coming in as well. They get to watch their friend or family member transform—looking and feeling ten to fifteen years younger within months.

> *Jayne: Age 52*
>
> *When I started this journey in 2017, I was 45 and didn't have any idea what was going on. I felt like I was too young to be going through menopause, but I didn't feel like myself at all. I was irritable for no reason, ravenous out of nowhere, and had horrible brain fog. I had absolutely zero interest in sex.*
>
> *My doctor did the usual bloodwork, assured me I was fine, and sent me on my way. Meanwhile, I felt like I was losing my mind. I was suffering, I knew something wasn't right, I figured it was hormones. But I didn't know who to go to.*

Thankfully, a friend of mine did hormone replacement therapy and suggested I give it a try.

I'm so grateful to have found Cunningham Clinic because I have a partner in this journey, helping me to get balanced and feel like myself again. It took some time to figure the right cocktail of hormones but I'm finally on the right path.

Now I send everyone in to get the bloodwork done. Knowledge is power. I could be the poster child for HRT, and I will tell anyone who will listen how much better I feel.

GET YOUR LABS CHECKED

Here are the minimum labs you should have checked to get started:
- CBC (complete blood count)
- CMP (comprehensive metabolic panel)
- Vitamin D (also called D-25 hydrox)
- Vitamin B_{12}
- Full thyroid panel including
  - ◊ TSH (thyroid stimulating hormone)
  - ◊ Free T3
  - ◊ Free or Total T4
  - ◊ TPO Antibodies
- Hemoglobin A1C
- Lipid panel
- PSA (men over 40)
- Total testosterone* (both men and women)
- Estradiol* (both men and women)
- Free testosterone* (both men and women)
- SHBG* (sex hormone binding globulin both men and women)
- FSH (follicle stimulating hormone) (women)
- LH (luteinizing hormone) (men)
- Prolactin (men)
- Ferretin (women)

*these labs should be completed using LCMS/MS Assay for accurate results

WHAT IS LCMS/MS ASSAY?

LabCorp, Access Medlabs, Quest and other lab companies are now able to offer hormone labs results utilizing Liquid Chromatography Mass Spectrometry (LCMS/MS Assay). This is a much more accurate and specific way to measure sex hormones and allows providers to tailor care to each specific client's original levels as well as how s/he responds to treatment. The old way of measuring hormones, called immunoassay, can be less accurate and many HRT providers are moving to LCMS/MS Assay for sex hormones for better patient outcomes.

WOMEN AND MENOPAUSE

Most clients come into my office with a familiar tale of misdiagnosed symptoms, having been told their symptoms are largely in their head, or like I was, to just need to *grin and bear* their symptoms of low energy, urinary incontinence, low sex drive etc., etc., as a natural part of the aging process.

I hear the following sentence every day, often more than once a day: *I feel awful, but no one can find anything wrong.*

Because most women are suffering from a combination of the various symptoms in varying degrees, and no two people are exactly alike, it's important to know what's behind the cascade of seemingly unrelated issues.

WHAT BODILY PROCESSES DO HORMONES AFFECT?

- Metabolism
- Growth and development
- Emotions and mood
- Fertility and sexual function
- Sleep
- Blood pressure
- Muscle development
- Bone and connective tissue health

PELVIC FLOOR CHANGES

A healthy pelvic floor, like that of a 30-year-old, is a nice, tight collection of muscles and ligaments that hold that pelvic floor, bladder, vaginal vault, and uterus in place.

As we age, testosterone levels drop. As a result, you lose muscle tone, and the pelvic floor can start to droop. When that happens, the rectus abdominis, which are the "six-pack" muscles and the transverse abdominis, which is the smiley face-shaped muscle between the belly button and the pubic bone, both begin to pooch.

Many people try to get the "easy fix" by going to get CoolSculpting® or liposuction. Others sign up for Pilates and yoga. They do every kind of exercise they can think of to get rid of that pooch, but the transverse abdominal muscle has just completely given out because it can't work without the pelvic floor supporting it. Unfortunately, without a healthy testosterone level, there's no way to build the blood vessels, nerve endings, and muscle tone required to pull that pelvic floor up, and then that transverse abdominis in. Women, in particular, spend all this time exercising in ways that can't ever make a difference because the basic building blocks aren't there.

The other unpleasant effect of a drop in testosterone is that as the pelvic floor atrophies and drops, the clitoris can become enveloped by that tissue. People think of atrophy as up and in, but the pelvic floor drops as it fails, and that's why the clitoris goes up into it. As the clitoris disappears, it's not as easily accessible. Because clitoral stimulus is integral to orgasmic achievement in women, and the clitoris can also lose nerve endings and blood supply due to low testosterone, that's going to change the quality and quantity of orgasms, depending on how much atrophy has occurred.

Simply stated, if you can't get to it, you can't stimulate it!

I was giving a talk once. While I was describing this absorption of the clitoris up and into the pelvic floor, a woman in the back of the room yelled out, "So, that's where it went!"

There was laughter, but also a lot of agreement.

URETHRAL ATROPHY

As the pelvic floor falls, the bladder wants to tilt because it's not being held up properly. As the bladder tilts, the urethra can become kinked which can also cause or increase urinary incontinence. This can affect all women, whether or not they have had children.

VAGINAL ATROPHY

A healthy vagina has really robust tissue thickness and secretory cells which produce moisture. At around age 50, the estrogen abates. As a result, the vaginal vault shortens and becomes thinner and more fragile from the lack of epithelial lining. The secretions stop, and no amount of lubrication is quite enough to stave off the dryness. Women describe sex as painful—like broken glass. Sometimes, there is bleeding. In addition, without estrogen, the external urethral sphincter gets atrophied and excoriated (roughed up and irritated). As a result, there can be both bladder leakage and a lot of irritation, which leads to an increase in the number of bladder infections and yeast infections.

LOSS OF MUSCLE TONE AND BONE DENSITY

When a woman doesn't have enough testosterone, she's not going to have enough muscle tone. Healthy, female adult testosterone levels on a blood test should be 80-250. When testosterone falls below 30 women usually can't grow muscle. Below 20, women usually can't grow bone, and that's called osteoporosis.

Humans develop muscle tissue by stressing the muscle or "working out." That process causes micro tears in the tissue stimulating growth as a response and, voila, bigger muscles and better tone. However, if a woman is working out really hard, determined to "get her body back" and her testosterone is below 30, she is actually getting fatter *faster* than her peers who aren't working out at all. All she is doing is breaking down the muscle tissue she has left and losing more and more strength with every trip to the gym.

It's a downright cruel reality.

HOT FLASHES

Sometimes you're driving, or you're in the middle of a meeting, or you're on a very important sales call, and suddenly you feel distracted and a little nauseous. A hot "flash" generally starts in the chest, goes up through the neck and exits out of the top of your head. For me, it felt like a million drops of lava were trying to escape out through my hair follicles, and I was surprised by how painful they were. Hot flashes are over in a minute, but it literally feels like you're about to spontaneously combust. You're left, shaky, pitted out, gross, and wondering what just happened.

Sometimes hot flashes are mixed up with night sweats, so I always have my clients describe how it feels. If a woman describes it as happening at night and waking up cold and in a puddle, that tells me it's a low testosterone issue, and they are having night sweats. Hot flashes are estrogen driven, typically short lived, very disruptive, sometimes painful, and they seem to come out of nowhere.

A hot flash happens when you don't have enough estrogen for whatever reason. So, in perimenopause, sometimes you'll ovulate on the right side, but not on the left. And sometimes, you'll ovulate two times on the left, and then not at all on the right. It's very much what I call popcorn style. It's all over the place, and it's really a pain. Hot flashes can happen once, or 20, even 30 times a day.

Women think that when hot flashes are over, they are through menopause, and they're all done, but the end of hot flashing only means their body got used to the estrogen withdrawal and now that they're at zero and no longer having these vasomotor symptoms. Unfortunately, without estrogen, you start getting fragile throughout the body. It's not just the vaginal vault that gets torn easily, but any of the skin gets very dry, wrinkly, and tears easily. Without estrogen, a woman's risks of Alzheimer's and heart disease go way up, so, this hormone is really important for longevity.

NIGHT SWEATS

In women, night sweats can begin when testosterone falls below 80 and can start up to 15 years before menopause because testosterone begins to drop at around age 35. Night sweats usually happen across the chest. You wake up and your shirt is soaking wet, and you don't know why. And then you're cold. Night sweats interrupt your sleep because you're changing your clothes two times a night and your sheets every day.

LOSS OF SLEEP

Sleep is multifactorial and really tricky, but when testosterone falls, many women start experiencing night sweats. When Vitamins D and B_{12} go down, women fall asleep or can't stay asleep. When thyroid gets low, sleep is disrupted as well. B_{12}, Vitamin D, thyroid, and hormones all contribute to sleep.

Estrogen is another complicating factor. When estrogen falls in a woman, cortisol goes up sky high. When cortisol goes up, the brain won't turn off and remains in constant stress mode. Women describe it like they are in perpetual fight or flight working toward an ever-moving finish line and just barely holding on. Life gets really hard when cortisol, aka stress, is driving the bus.

Also, when cortisol goes high, women deposit fat around the belly. So, not only has that transverse abdominis failed, but now they're depositing fat like crazy in the belly, and women start looking pregnant.

When you are in chronic stress—or sympathetic nervous system hyperstimulation mode—you wake up with nonexistent cortisol and start the caffeine. The caffeine stimulates a falsely high cortisol load, and has you craving sugar like crazy, making you crash even more. You pepper both throughout the day to manage energy. Your cortisol will spike at 7:00 p.m., and the only thing that feels good is a glass of wine and a slice of cake.

Not a great recipe for sleep.

FATIGUE

If you have no muscle tone, you're not sleeping at night, you haven't had sex in six months, everything hurts, and you need a nap to get ready for your nap because your thyroid and your testosterone are toast—you're going to be fatigued.

The other thing about fatigue is, because the testosterone and/or estrogen has/have fallen, and cortisol is running the show and you're in constant fight or flight, it is exhausting. You can never get "there" and it's mentally demoralizing to boot.

Let's say the stars align. You have a perfect week. You finally get to where you think you can take a nap and pass out for that stolen 20 minutes or even an hour. Without your hormones, you still don't recover. You wake up on Monday, and it's the same body that still isn't working. And now, that fatigue feels even heavier.

Without hormones, it's the kind of tired that hurts. You feel like you need a nap that lasts for a week. You need your blankie, and it's still not enough. It feels like it's in your bones. It's in your soul.

DEPRESSION

Depression, like sleep, is multifactorial. Some people simply have a predisposition for depression and need to be referred to a trusted psychiatric practitioner. However, there are independent risk factors for depression that include: testosterone below 80, Vitamin D below 70, and a Free T3 level below 3.5. When people come in on multiple mood stabilizers and I check their labs, if I discover they have a Vitamin D of 19, a testosterone of 0, and a free T3 of 1.5, I have no idea if they're depressed (as defined by a lack of neurotransmitters), but they most certainly have three correctable lab values that are each independent risk factors for depression. It is entirely possible they don't need those mood stabilizers but a different approach to addressing symptoms of depression.

Interestingly, the most common years for a woman to be prescribed an antidepressant are between ages 40 and 50. Whether or not there is a clinical depression must be investigated, but there is most certainly perimenopause/menopause at play. Perhaps that is why so many women in that age group are "poor responders" to antidepressants.

Somebody who says, "I've been on an antidepressant since I was 20," probably isn't coming off of their medication because they have a true serotonin or norepinephrine deficiency. When someone tells me they were fine until about age 37 and then it all went downhill, it can be a different story. It's classic to have someone who comes in on an antidepressant that they've been ratcheting up dosage-wise from where they started in their late 30s or early 40s. What we keep finding in my practice is what they had was a testosterone deficiency, never a serotonin deficiency or a norepinephrine deficiency.

In a perfect scenario, I can start checking women at around age 35 because testosterone starts to fall 15 years before menopause, which is at an average age of 50.

WEIGHT GAIN

"Five years ago, all I had to do was take a couple of laps around the park, and I could fit into my jeans. Now, I eat 500 calories a day, and I'm gaining weight."

Sound familiar?

As we age, weight gain is another multifactorial condition. In the absence of estrogen, cortisol increases and leads to fat deposition on the stomach. By age 45, 50% or more of Americans do not make deiodinase (that's the enzyme required to cut the T4 your thyroid produces into Free T3—the active part). So, even though their TSH is normal, they do not have a functioning thyroid system. Weight gain in women is further complicated when testosterone falls below 30. Motivated women who are serious about losing weight go to Orange Theory® or join a CrossFit® gym and start working out like crazy. It makes sense, right?

Not so fast . . .

When you work out, you're supposed to be breaking down your muscle fibers to build up bigger, stronger, better muscles. But when you don't have testosterone, all you can do is break down muscle that you cannot build back up. And the volume of muscles in the body makes up the resting metabolic rate.

The more you work without testosterone, the more you are replacing muscle with connective tissue and fat. When you don't have muscle, you don't have a resting metabolic rate. So now, instead of 1200 to 1500 calories to be alive as a human, maybe you only need 800 or 900. That is a sad day in the kitchen when you are limited to 800 calories or you gain weight, right?

Without a functioning thyroid, you don't have any active metabolism either. You're working out but you have no muscle tone, and the resting metabolic rate is in the toilet. So, you think about a slice of cake, and that's five pounds.

Absent both a functioning thyroid system and enough testosterone, you're just going to start packing on the pounds, and it snowballs in almost a logarithmic scale. It's a little bit, a little bit more, and then, suddenly, it's a lot.

INFLAMMATION, PAIN, AND DISEASE

Pain is inflammation. Most of the diseases of aging are diseases of inflammation. If you look at type 2 diabetes, cancer, heart disease, bad cholesterol, high blood pressure, arthritis, and pain, they all include inflammatory processes. Without testosterone, autoimmune processes go way up because testosterone is actually the most powerful anti-inflammatory you can put in a human being. As we get older and our testosterone falls, we're increasingly fragile and constantly in an inflammatory state.

LOSS OF LIBIDO

You are losing pelvic floor muscle tone. It hurts to have sex, and you have urinary leakage. You suffer hot flashes and night sweats. Even if you didn't battle both fatigue and insomnia, the extra 15 pounds you've gained and your chronic pain have you feeling anything but sexy. Never mind your clitoris seems to have moved.

While your partner might miss intimacy with you enough to brave the puddle of sweat on your side of the bed, you feel anything but sexy. It's a recipe for physical and marital disaster.

In a nutshell, you've lost sex drive because your estrogen and testosterone has fallen off.

In the next chapters we will examine how to solve this complex constellation of issues with treatments that work.

> ***Ann: Age 60***
>
> *I remember going into the gynecologist's office at age 53. I hadn't slept for six months—like not slept. She looked at me and said, "You look terrible."*
>
> *"Well, yeah," I said. "I just haven't slept."*
>
> *I was having terrible hot flashes. And it wasn't just like I got hot, it was a raging kind of a feeling. I've never been an emotional person and I would be feeling like I was going to cry. I was losing track of things. It was not good.*
>
> *My sex life was worse. I was never really interested. I was going along with it and I never said no but we were raising three rambunctious, crazy boys, I was working full-time and I was just so tired.*

How Do You Feel?

A Checklist For Women to Assess for Hormone Deficiency

- *Extreme* fatigue
- Hitting a wall between three and four p.m.
- Mood swings
- Anxiety
- Tension & irritability
- Lack of sleep
- Wake up at three to four a.m.
- Memory loss
- Depression
- Lack of focus
- Brain fog
- Hot flashes
- Night sweats
- Weight gain
- Joint pain
- Bladder symptoms
- Migraine/severe headache
- Decreased sex drive and/or performance

HORMONE REPLACEMENT THERAPY FOR WOMEN

The most common misconception I hear from women is, "I'm done with menopause. I don't need hormones because I'm not symptomatic anymore."

I always respond with the same question. "How's your sex life?"

Despite the surprise, a familiar expression crosses their face. The honest answers I get range from, "I'm fine with a tube of lube, a couple of glasses of wine, and a vibrator," to, "It takes so long, it's not even worth having an orgasm, because I've got to find the spot and then, by the time I actually get to orgasm, I've run through ten different fantasies in my head and my partner's exhausted." Many women admit they tell their partners they are good or pretend they had an orgasm because it's just not worth it to get there.

Just because you're done having hot flashes, it doesn't mean you don't need hormones. And some women have hot flashes on and off indefinitely. We need estrogen for the skin, so it doesn't tear every time we just brush against the wall, for our faces to be less wrinkly, and for the heart and brain to stay intact. We need estrogen for the vaginal vault. Without it, micro tears occur with the introduction of a penis, toy, or sexual activity, and women have a painful sandpapery feeling that is antithetical to orgasm.

One client told me that the estrogen in her HRT saved her marriage. Sex with her husband was so painful, they simply weren't having any. They were basically roommates until she got on HRT.

The only women who can't receive estrogen are women with a history of epilepsy (unless their neurologist says it's okay) and women with an estrogen-positive cancer—either currently or previously. I have many clients who have been cleared by oncology to keep getting their estrogen, and that's fine. It's just a conversation to coordinate with other care providers.

Testosterone, on the other hand, is generally safe for *all* women, and we need it for so much more.

Men aged 30-70 will lose 10% testosterone production per year
Women aged 20-40 lose up to 50% testosterone production per year!

PELVIC FLOOR IMPROVEMENTS WITH HRT

Some women have an interesting reaction soon after starting hormone replacement therapy. There's a week or two in the beginning where they can't wear jeans because the stiff material can be stimulating. It's a little uncomfortable and maybe even distracting. This is due to the pelvic floor starting to tighten back up which corrects clitoral positioning, improved uterine orientation, and releases pressure on the urethra.

The sensation they feel is expected and normal, if a bit unexpected.

WEIGHT LOSS AND IMPROVED MUSCLE TONE

Initially, weight gain is from a drop in hormones and, often, a thyroid imbalance, so people think getting their hormone levels up means the uptick in weight will come right off. Unfortunately, it's not that simple. Perimenopausal hormone fat on women is sticky fat, and it takes extra work to get it off.

Because so many women have been trained to be slaves to the scale, I tell all my clients, the first thing they're going to do on HRT is gain weight because they are rebuilding muscle, muscle weighs more than fat (not really, a pound is a pound of course. It's just that a pound of fat is about the size of a six-inch sub sandwich and a pound of muscle is smaller than your fist), and new muscle likes to hold onto water. My biggest and best advice is, "Stay off the scale for the first three months!"

Women will put on about five to seven pounds on average, and that's a good thing, because with the muscles, the pelvic floor is going to lift and the transverse abdominis is coming back. With more muscle, the resting metabolic rate increases. As soon as the hormones are replaced and they are all balanced, they can go back to the gym or do whatever workout regimen they like, and then the weight begins to come off.

FIXING NIGHT SWEATS

Testosterone—pure and simple.

BETTER SLEEP

If your testosterone levels are low, sleep disturbances increase. If your sleep is disturbed, you can't reach REM sleep where your body produces testosterone.

While that is the very definition of a vicious cycle, getting your testosterone levels back to normal helps with the synchronization and helps to lower cortisol levels. From there, we can start fixing all of the things that are wrong. Sleep takes about six months to really get dialed back in. Sometimes, I have to put clients on different supplements, and it's typically a multi-step process. When you aren't waking up soaking wet, you sleep through the night. When you start feeling better and aren't a sweaty mess, you feel sexier and orgasms help you sleep better etc., etc., so every step feeds into the next.

LESS FATIGUE

One of the immediate benefits of testosterone is a boost in energy. I have yet to put anyone on HRT who hasn't commented on how much more energetic they feel, or how they've given up that afternoon nap they felt like they had to have.

DEPRESSION HELP

It takes about a year, depending on how many mood stabilizers someone is on to start peeling away the medications in order to see what's underneath. More than half the time, the people on antidepressants who see me are not actually depressed, they're just endocrinologically deficient.

The first thing is NOT to have a client stop taking any of the medications prescribed by the other health professionals they see. I've got to bring the base up first and get the body functioning to see: if they are actually depressed, it truly is a hormone imbalance, or both. If I can fix the biology, then we start to wean them off what they are taking, slowly, with coordinated medical supervision.

I also recommend exercise. Exercise gives you endorphins. When you are balanced hormonally you can move your body. When you can have sex, exercise, and do all the things that make you happy, symptoms of depression tend to diminish or resolve.

REDUCING OSTEOPOROSIS

The primary medication for osteoporosis is called a bisphosphonate. The best remineralization it can get you is about 2% a year, and that's only the outer shell of the bone. So, if you fall, your risk of fracture is just about the same, and that medication can cause jaw tumors and other bad side effects, such as esophageal erosions.

When testosterone is replaced, your bone mineralization can increases up to 8.5% every year. And that's the outer shell as well as that inner malleable part of the bone. If you trip and fall, but have better bone density and stronger muscles that can catch you, there's a better chance you won't break anything. As you age, you can function in your daily life with some protection.

REDUCED INFLAMMATION, PAIN, AND DISEASE

Testosterone is the most powerful anti-inflammatory you can put in a man or a woman. The end. There is nothing stronger than testosterone to prevent inflammation.

Autoimmune disease is a condition of inflammation and immunity. By some studies, if you've had one uncontrolled autoimmune disease your risk of getting another is 75-85% in the next five to ten years. By the time someone comes into the clinic, they sometimes have multiple autoimmune diagnoses to deal with. In order to support them best I can, we assess what their needs are on multiple fronts including Vitamin D, and other supplements. If I push the testosterone a bit higher than I normally would, it often quiets those autoimmune processes and even gets them to go dormant. While testosterone isn't a cure, I can get some people off some of the immune suppressive drugs they are taking.

What we have seen in the bioidentical hormone replacement world is consistent with the hypothesis that if you reduce the inflammatory state, you reduce the risk of a host of diseases and illnesses. Breast cancer is definitely a disease of inflammation, and HRT that included testosterone was shown in 2022 in the study mentioned above to DECREASE the risk of breast cancer by about 38% and the risk of invasive breast cancer by almost 59%. Why? You have natural killer cells and T cells, and you have an immune system that's designed to break down cancer and make better cells. It's called autophagy. But when you've got solid tumors starting to grow, and your immune system can't stay ahead of that, it becomes a solid tumor cancer—breast cancer, pancreatic cancer, etc.

With the combination of testosterone and regular checkups, as well as a mammogram, pelvic ultrasound, and a colonoscopy, the preventative health clinician in me feels confident I'm doing all I can to ensure the best health for all of my clients.

SEXY TIMES AHEAD

One of my more gratifying experiences as a health care provider has been working with a stunningly beautiful client I'll call Stacy. Stacy was 55 when she came in for the first time. She'd gone through menopause ten years earlier with no hormone support since that time from any of her providers.

I have no idea how she even made it to get to me because her numbers on all fronts were terrible. Her Vitamin D was at 19. Her free T3 was at 1.5 and she had zero testosterone and estrogen. I developed a recovery program for her to start feeling better, and she started right away. At the four-month mark, she came in to see me, and her levels had all risen into normal ranges.

"You know, I want to have sex all the time, but I don't have a boyfriend," she told me.

"You weren't likely to have a boyfriend before because you weren't emitting a single pheromone, and you were just so shut down that you probably weren't even going to make a new friend, let alone somebody to have sex with," I told her. "Now, you're not only gorgeous but putting out into the world that you're available."

She was engaged six months later.

Testosterone for the win!

Vickey: Age 58

I was working as a consultant in a predominantly male dominated industry (transportation and oil and gas) when I started having hot flashes. Sitting in a conference room with a dozen managers and engineers (mostly guys) while I was flashing was crazy. I just wanted to rip all of my clothes off and run screaming down the hallway. Maintaining composure and concentration was difficult to say the least. Thanks to hormones, I saved my sanity, my mind, my reputation, and my career.

> **Ann: Age 60**
>
> *Literally within five days of starting hormone replacement therapy I began to feel like myself again. I started sleeping through the night. Gone went a lot of the brain fog that was a function of not sleeping. My menopausal symptoms improved. It was crazy how much better I felt.*
>
> *I have friends who don't want to have sex anymore. I have a friend whose anxiety and emotions are all over the place. Others are depressed. "Try this," I tell them. "It will make your life better."*
>
> *I swear I tell everyone.*

POSITIVE EFFECTS OF NATURAL TESTOSTERONE FOR MEN & WOMEN

- Increased energy, vitality & zest for life
- Improved feeling of overall well-being
- Depression relief
- Anxiety relief
- Improved cognitive clarity
- Improved memory
- Improved focus
- Prostate protection
- Breast protection
- Cardiovascular protection
- Increased bone strength
- Increased muscle strength
- Reduced body fat
- Lower cholesterol
- Enhanced libido
- Enhanced performance

POSITIVE EFFECTS OF NATURAL ESTROGEN FOR WOMEN

- Improved mood
- No more hot flashes
- Vaginal health and juiciness
- Brain protection against Alzheimer's
- Heart protection against heart disease
- Lower cortisol levels
- Help get rid of belly fat
- Great looking skin

MEN AND MIDDLE AGE

Like women, men also begin to experience "olditis," and it's all in the numbers.

A healthy adult male's testosterone should be 900 to 1,100 and elite athletes can go a little higher, as high as 1,450.

Below 900, the risk of Alzheimer's in men goes up by as much as 40%. Although it's a disease that typically affects women more than men, that's a huge jump in risk.

Below 700, the prostate can start to enlarge, and there is an increased risk of prostate cancer. Further complicating the situation, an enlarged prostate can pinch off the urethra. Flomax and Avodart, the medications most commonly prescribed to help empty a man's bladder can cause erectile dysfunction. Viagra® is then prescribed so those men can pee and have sex. I hate it when I see someone who is caught up in this scenario, when we may have been able to prevent this by keeping the testosterone from falling too low in the first place.

Below 600, all-cause mortality goes up sixfold. It's not entirely clear why, but men just die six times more often than their same aged peers when they have a testosterone lower than 600.

Below 500 there is an increased risk of obesity, diabetes, heart disease, high blood pressure, bad cholesterol, arthritis, and any of the diseases of inflammation, including cancer. Not to mention increased pain, crappy sleep, and loss of muscle tone.

Below 300 (and by some insurances and practice groups below 287, which seems like a very arbitrary number) men will often have abject erectile dysfunction—meaning a man will not be able to have an erection that is sustainable for long enough to complete a sexual encounter. At this point, he may, finally, be offered testosterone. That is a long way to fall before a provider will do something about such an easily remedied issue.

In men, testosterone levels start to fall around age 35 and really begin to drop off by age 50. Ideally, he should start checking around age 35 to avoid sliding through those risk strata and avoid any time at higher risk by not having enough testosterone.

FACTS ABOUT ANDROPAUSE

- 20% of males over 50 have low testosterone by American standards. The percentage is much higher by other standards.
- Common in men with diabetes, high BP, sleep apnea & other chronic disease
- Linked to early heart disease
- Underdiagnosed

PELVIC FLOOR CHANGES

Similar to women, as a man loses muscle tone, his pelvic floor drops. When testosterone and thyroid fall, men will often start to develop a fat deposition between their belly button and their penis. The transverse abdominis also fails in the man, and the rectus abdominis becomes floppy. Now, the lower abdominal wall is pushing forward, and fat deposits on top of that. As a result, the penis can be pulled up into the lower abdomen and appear to lose length.

ERECTILE DYSFUNCTION

If a man is not experiencing regular morning erections, that is one measure of erectile dysfunction. Time to subsequent encounter is another measure of sexual wellness. When you're 15, you might need 15 minutes of rest and you're ready to go again. When you're 50, twice in one day might be a bit ambitious. The longer and longer it takes to recover enough to have a subsequent encounter is also a measure of erectile dysfunction. Other measures of erectile dysfunction include the number of erections per week, difficulty getting an erection, having erections that are not hard enough for penetration, unsatisfactory intercourse, loss of erection after penetration, loss of sexual interest and desire, and ejaculatory strength.

When men are single for a year or two years, and they don't have many or any sexual encounters, masturbatory efforts are typically more easily achieved even in the presence of erectile dysfunction, because they can control stimulus, thought process, and pressure. When they go back to having sex with someone else, they often realize they don't have enough strength to complete the encounter with another human.

"Something has happened," they will tell me.

My answer is often, "Over the last two to three years, as your testosterone fell, so did blood flow."

Loss of testosterone is one of the primary culprits behind erectile dysfunction.

SYMPTOMS OF ERECTILE DYSFUNCTION

- Difficulty getting an erection
- Difficulty maintaining an erection long enough for sexual intimacy
- Having erections that are not hard enough for penetration
- Unsatisfactory intercourse

LOSS OF MUSCLE TONE

The numbers aren't as hard and fixed with men, but at a testosterone level below 600, most men struggle to grow muscle. Eventually, the shoulders start to slope and the head starts to come forward. That hunchbacked, sloped shoulder is a clear sign of not enough testosterone for an extended period of time. As the back and stomach muscles atrophy a man's belly comes forward, the butt loses projection, and a fat pad forms that hides the penis. Sometimes there's actually gynecomastia (male breast development), an unpleasant side effect of weight gain. Because fat makes its own estrogen, there is an increased risk of a man developing more breast tissue.

LOSS OF LIBIDO

When testosterone falls below 80, most women simply lose the urge to have sex. With men it's more complicated but estimated to be at around 500 or 550. We know that as testosterone falls, men start to lose interest in sex or finding a partner.

In women, a drop in libido manifests as an *I'm too tired,* or *I don't want to.* In men it's a little bit murkier. It might be that there's actually some measures of erectile dysfunction they're trying to avoid. Men tend to avoid poor performance—on the football field, in the boardroom, in the bedroom—it's a coping mechanism.

But, boy, they certainly tell me all about it when their sex drive and ability to perform comes back. They're very happy!

One of my clients told me he hadn't dated for a long time and wasn't lonely. It just didn't occur to him to try and go out and meet someone or get onto a dating site. After we got him on testosterone and feeling good, he told me that if he had started sooner, he might not have all these cats!

LOSS OF SLEEP

As testosterone falls, sleep quality decreases. Men don't typically get night sweats, but they will have problems falling asleep or staying asleep. When a man is not sleeping through the night regularly, he will often gain weight. In fact, insomnia is usually responsible for about ten pounds all by itself. If we can fix sleep in a man, they can usually get those ten pounds right back off in less than six months.

DEPRESSION

When testosterone falls, mood disorders go up. The number one age for a man to be prescribed an antidepressant is age 45 to 55. A drop in testosterone clearly equals an increase in depression and anxiety, especially when his sexual performance is impacted. The double insult of low testosterone and antidepressants can radically impact a man's sex drive and his ability to complete the act.

WEIGHT GAIN

Men gain weight for multiple reasons. One is poor sleep, two is loss of muscle tone which affects resting metabolic rate. Because of low testosterone and, often, thyroid, the resting metabolic rate drops and weight increases. In men, there is a loss of desire to exercise in this situation because they are achy, and they don't feel great when they're done working out. I have found that men will avoid exercise sooner than women, and I suspect it goes back to avoiding poor performance as a coping mechanism. If a man can't work out or lift like he used to, he will often avoid the activity entirely.

INCREASED RISK OF DISEASES OF INFLAMMATION

Testosterone is the most powerful anti-inflammatory you can put in a human, male or female. Without natural anti-inflammatories, anything that's driven by inflammation, is, of course, going to get worse and worse. That's one of the reasons why these are diseases of aging. As the testosterone falls, all these bad things start to go up. While it is a correlation, not a causation, the data shows the risk of cancer goes up, risk of diabetes goes up, heart disease, high blood pressure, cholesterol issues, arthritis, and even gout increase at a testosterone level around 400.

INCREASED PAIN

From twisting your ankle to getting dental work—everything just hurts more because testosterone is your natural anti-inflammatory.

BRAIN FOG IN MEN

That feeling of confusion, forgetfulness, lack of focus and mental clarity, otherwise known as brain fog, is caused by testosterone and thyroid deficiencies. It is especially noticeable in the afternoon. Men report to me that they prefer to schedule morning meetings and not be available later in the day, knowing they won't be at their best.

FATIGUE

Fatigue is a big symptom of low testosterone in men as well as women. If somebody wants a nap every single day, that's a pretty good sign that they have no or low testosterone, and probably no or low thyroid functionality. A lot of men will tell me they are planning for retirement, stopping their sport, or they are planning to have more rest time. After they start hormone replacement therapy, all that's out the window. I get started with them and usually within a year, they are a very different person—back to their sport, they are doing something else with their company, or they are going after a new pursuit. It's really fun to watch the change from the guy who sort of slunk or skulked in with an unhappy face and a list of complaints transition back into being a virile, functioning adult full of excitement for what they can do again.

Some clients are fast responders, and then some are what I call a "slow burn" and take a few rounds of pellets to really start to feel better. My husband was one of the slow burners. I checked his levels immediately when starting Cunningham Clinic and was surprised to find he was in the 500s given he didn't have any outward symptoms. I started him on pellets, and then realized it turned out he was symptomatic after all. Right around the ninth month on hormone replacement therapy, my husband was delighted to see that he had lost four inches off his waist and many of his dress shirts were too small in the biceps. Even more impressive was the return of his performance on the bike. My husband has always been an avid cyclist but had, as many do, slowed down a bit on his cycling stamina. Slowing down in one's sport is absolutely a sign of low or falling testosterone levels and does *not* have to be "normal." Right around that ninth month on hormone replacement therapy, he hopped on his mountain bike and climbed over 3000 vertical feet without stopping. He realized he was training almost every single day, feeling as robust as he did in grad school and enjoying having the appetite to go with it.

Jason: Age 52

My wife went into Cunningham Clinic, started HRT, and I saw how great she looked and felt. After doing a little bit more research on the safety and efficacy for men, I decided to make an appointment for myself to talk over philosophies, testing, and a game plan. I decided to go with it and it's been nothing but amazing for both of us.

As a man, there is absolutely no reason not to get your blood drawn for low testosterone. There is no shame in finding out you can take a life-changing step to improve the way you feel.

You can look at your levels and then make an educated, knowledgeable decision about what is best for you and your partner.

I experienced a steady and noticeable improvement in energy at the gym, work, and even at the end of the day. My brain fog disappeared and my mood improved. As you can imagine, that led to better performance in the bedroom.

Men who are resistant to such positive improvement are just missing out. They really are. I've talked to several people about being on hormone replacement and discovered I'm definitely not alone. No one who is on it regrets their decision.

I just wish I had started sooner.

Mike: Age 76

Am I glad I started HRT at Cunningham Clinic? You bet your booties I am because it's given me a new outlook on life. It's enabled me to become more athletic and healthier. Will I continue to do it? Yes, I will, probably until you put the nail in the coffin. It's increased my health, it's increased my ability to recover from knee and other surgeries I've had since I've been on the therapy. And so, yes, it's fantastic.

I know how I feel and I know that I feel great when I'm on the therapy. And I also know that as my time on the therapy starts to expire I can tell that I'm regressing back to my old, pre-therapy physical situation. It's like it's running out and I need to re-dose.

It makes 76 year-old-me feel like, well, maybe not a 40-year-old but definitely a 50-year-old. I'm still doing the same things that I did before therapy, but I'm doing them in a healthier and pain free manner.

I'm so glad that we got introduced to it and we tell all of our friends and neighbors. Some of them take advantage of it, some of them don't. The ones who don't—well that's their loss.

How Do You Feel?
A Checklist For Men to Assess for Hormone Deficiency

- *Extreme* fatigue
- Hitting a wall between three and four p.m.
- Mood swings
- Anxiety
- Tension & irritability
- Lack of sleep
- Memory loss
- Decline in stamina
- Depression
- Lack of focus
- Brain fog
- Weight gain
- Loss of muscle tone
- Joint pain
- Erectile dysfunction/loss of erectile strength
- Bladder problems/frequent urination
- Decreased sex drive and/or performance
- Not as interested/competent in physical activity

OTHER HORMONES MATTER

H*ow do you feel? How is your body functioning?*
I ask everyone these crucial questions, but especially people who tell me, "Oh, my doctor did my labs, I'm fine."

"Print them out, give them to me," I always tell them.

Often, what I get is a CBC, and a chemistry, and a cholesterol. That's it. No hormones, no vitamin levels, and no thyroid. Maybe they got a TSH, but they didn't do the whole panel for thyroid and they didn't get a Vitamin D or a B_{12}. My lab panel, which currently costs $200, tells a much more complete picture.

There are over 2,000 known endocrine disruptors (chemical additives) in the United States, starting from the BPA in the plastic bottles to the federally mandated flame retardant that was added into children's pajamas for over a decade. We are constantly being attacked by endocrine (hormone) disruptors in the United States and endocrine disrupting food. Farming practices in the U.S. over the last 50 or so years have maximized crop yield at the expense of nutritional content, and we don't have enough *food* in our food to even support our bodies, let alone undo the damage from these endocrine disruptors.

One food example is Diindolylmethane, or DIM for short, which is what makes broccoli and other cruciferous vegetables superfoods. In the 1940s and 1950s, we ate a serving of broccoli or Brussels sprouts, and we had our daily supply of DIM. In the United States today, women have to have about 20 servings of broccoli and men have to have up to 40 servings of broccoli to get enough diindolylmethane.

Women are definitely more affected than men by hormone disruptors, probably because of the cosmetics we use, which can be a huge delivery mechanism of endocrine disruptors. If it says "phthalate" or "fragrance" on the label, there's a pretty good chance it's an endocrine disruptor. And women like to soak in it. We get our Epsom salt bath with our extra lavender, and if it's not a real essential oil, then it could have something in it that isn't good for us.

Because we are being attacked from birth with chemicals that prevent the body from being able to manufacture hormones and the nutrients in our food nutrients are greatly diminished, I not only check for testosterone and estrogen in menopausal women, and testosterone in men, but Vitamins D and B_{12} and the full scope of thyroid function for everyone.

HORMONES AT-A-GLANCE

- Hormone imbalance can occur in men and women at any age
- Not all therapies are equal
- Hormone balance is not a "one size fits all" approach
- Low, "normal" labs may not be **_Optimal_** *(Vitamin D_3, Thyroid, Testosterone, B_{12}, etc.)*

THYROID

It is estimated that about 50% of the population over the age of 50 in the United States has what's called low Free T3 syndrome.

Symptomatic women experience fatigue, weight gain, hair loss, dry skin, cold intolerance, depression, and brittle nails. Symptomatic men experience the same issues, but the weight gain tends to be around the waistline. low Free T3 syndrome occurs when the thyroid functionality starts to wane because of the decrease in deiodinase production. One of my male clients described the change in his physique to me as, "An inner tube around my middle I definitely don't need. I already know how to swim; the last thing I need is a built in floatie!"

Here's how this overcomplicated system works: The thyroid is a gland in your neck that makes what's called T4. Out in your body, you make two different enzymes called deiodinase one and deiodinase two, which "cut" or convert T4 down into Free T3. Between these two thyroid hormones, it is important to know that T4 is, essentially, a potential or parent compound, and then Free T3 is the active or functional compound. For the system to work, T4 must be converted or cut into Free T3. This is why Free T3 is your metabolism, your hair quality and quantity, your brain clarity, the ability to regulate temperature, and more.

Your brain then reads the sum total of all thyroid hormone derivatives, T4, T3, T2, and T1, as one lump amount, which prompts the production of TSH, which "tells" the thyroid gland to make more T4. If you don't make deiodinase one or two anymore, you can have plenty of T4, but your Free T3 is nonexistent. That means while there is nothing wrong with your thyroid gland itself, your system out in the body is not working and you are still experiencing symptoms of hypothyroidism. Primary hypothyroidism, as defined by a high TSH lab value, means the *thyroid* is broken. Low Free T3 syndrome, as defined by a low Free T3 lab value, means the *system* is broken.

Medical professionals in the United States are really good about getting a TSH every year as part of an annual panel. Unfortunately, a basic TSH test only tells you whether or not the thyroid has finally gotten so bad the brain has noticed. By the time the TSH is high, the Free T3 has often been low for as much as ten to even 20 years.

If a provider is only getting the TSH, he or she has no idea if the system is working or if it is broken. So, what happens in a "regular" doctor's office when someone goes in with all the symptoms of low thyroid and all that is checked is a TSH which comes back "normal" the endocrinologist or the primary care provider will say they're fine.

Clients often just walk away, frustrated and without an answer. Meanwhile, the client has put on weight, is losing hair, can't think their way out of a cardboard box, and is depressed and cranky.

I get a Total T4 or a Free T4 *and* a Free T3 so I can prove that the conversion rate isn't happening. I really don't care as much about the TSH. I treat to the Free T3 because that's the functional part of an adult's thyroid system. I check antibodies as well. Because if you're making antibodies against your thyroid, you have an autoimmune disease called Hashimoto's Thyroiditis. Some big hospital groups don't check this because having positive thyroid antibodies do not increase the risk of thyroid cancer. And that's true. They don't. However, if you have one autoimmune disease that's out of control, your risk of getting a second or third in the next five to ten years is 75% by some studies. I don't want anyone to get Multiple Sclerosis, or Lupus, or Crohn's disease, or any of these other really bad autoimmune diseases. I want to make sure that's not going on and I want to catch Hashimoto's thyroiditis early and get it under control before any more autoimmune conditions join the party.

Another often missed lab is Ferritin. Ferritin is from iron and is the final transport molecule that takes the Free T3 into the cell to actually work. You can have a functioning thyroid, a functioning deiodinase/conversion system and *still* be clinically hypothyroid because you can't get the hormone into the cell. It's important to measure all of the components of a system to make sure you know where the system needs fixing.

I got into an argument once with an endocrinologist. His client, a 35 year-old female, came to me for a consult. Her hair was falling out in clumps and she couldn't stop crying. Her TSH was low or "corrected" because he'd given her enough Synthroid, a thyroid medication that only contains T4, but she'd put on nearly 15 pounds. I did bloodwork and discovered she actually had plenty of testosterone so perimenopause wasn't her issue, but her total T4, which should be around 8, and her free T3 which should be around 4, was 15:1. She wasn't making deiodinase so she couldn't cut her medication into active thyroid anymore. What used to work fine when she was younger was no longer the right medication.

I switched her from synthetic T4, which is Synthroid or levothyroxine, to a combination medication called NP Thyroid, that is T3 and T4 combined at the ratio that's required at the cellular level. Her hair grew back, she lost the weight, she stopped crying, and she went off the antidepressant she'd been taking.

That's when the argument happened. Her doctor called and began to yell at me.

"You can't change my client's prescription," he said.

"Oh, I can," I said. "In fact, why don't I have her sign a release of information and I'll fax you the labs. I can prove what the problem was and how it's being fixed."

My client, who feels great, and now has a full head of hair, will never go back to that endocrinologist.

VITAMIN D

Vitamin D actually functions as a hormone in the human body. We need Vitamin D for our immune system and for sleep. When Vitamin D falls, depression and anxiety can increase. When Vitamin D is really low, the thyroid often doesn't work properly either.

Decades ago, studies published in the *British Medical Journal* concluded that a Vitamin D level above 70 reduced the severity of autoimmune diseases, allergies, and asthma by as much as 70%.

Low Vitamin D in children looks like ADHD. Low Vitamin D over the age of 65 looks like Alzheimer's type dementia. Because both of these conditions typically are diagnoses of examination, as in there's not a blood test for it, not checking Vitamin D first can cause some confusion in properly determining the true condition.

20 years ago, I worked in skilled nursing facilities. When someone fell and broke something, I'd order a Vitamin D test. Almost always, the person's level would be 19 or even lower. At the time, I couldn't even get the test covered by Medicare or Medicaid unless the patient had a history of falls. Today, people still aren't getting Vitamin D but they're diagnosing ADHD without getting any bloodwork. Maybe it is ADHD, but since I didn't go to magic school, I believe it's crucial to check. In the elderly, clients are often diagnosed with Alzheimer's type dementia because the client fails a three-word recall or a mini-mental status exam. I want to know what's going on with the Vitamin D, the thyroid, and the testosterone before I'll diagnose anything.

Even though Vitamin D is called the sunshine vitamin, most people do not synthesize Vitamin D properly anymore. People come in telling me they are at the pool every day and their Vitamin D is in the low twenties. Even though they're tan that doesn't mean they're making Vitamin D. Of the 2,000 known endocrine disruptors in the United States, one of them is sunscreen. You put your sunscreen on so you won't need so much Botox, but unfortunately it's going to block your vitamin D production.

Interestingly enough, about ten years ago, Finland did a study where they gave one group of newborns 1,000 units a day of Vitamin D for their first year of life. Type 1 diabetes risk went down by 90% in that group.

When someone is Vitamin D deficient, I give them either 5,000 or 10,000 units of Vitamin D combined with 500 units of A and 500 units of K in one little pill. Vitamins A and K serve to open the door to get the D in the body. Because Vitamin D is a fat-soluble vitamin, it needs to be taken with food that contains fat in order to be absorbed—cheese, meat products, even coffee with creamer. Taken together, these three supplements will actually improve Vitamin D levels pretty quickly.

I had a client in her early thirties come in for a screening, and her chief complaint was that she thought something was horribly wrong. She had seen her primary care provider, a psychiatrist, and an endocrinologist who all told her there was "nothing wrong." She had extreme fatigue, poor mood, and felt that her concentration ability was just gone. Her labs all looked great by my standards except for one – her Vitamin D was at 10. *TEN!* That is critically low, and we started her with a shot of Vitamin D followed by an aggressive replacement protocol. Within three months all of her symptoms had resolved, she felt amazing, and she sent in all of her coworkers for a screening.

B_{12}

When people are dragging, they will get a B_{12} shot. When they drink too much, or if they feel like they're coming down with something, they go get a B_{12} shot.

Why?

Because B vitamins are your energy.

B_{12}, B_6, and Folic Acid are the big three. Low B_{12} is associated with depression and anxiety, low B_6 is associated with major depression and anxiety, and low folic acid is associated with anemia.

I only need to measure B_{12} in my lab tests because all of the B vitamins go together. I know if one's low, they're all low and I'll replace them with a combination product containing B_{12}, folic acid, and B_6 all at the same time. It makes a huge difference. The B_{12} reference range for one of the two major labs in the United States is 212 to 1,200—a 1000 point spread, which just once again shows the ridiculously unhelpful printout that is the "reference range." For my clients, the goal is 700 to 1,000 because when your B_{12} is 700 to 1,000, you actually have some energy. You have the ability to plan and execute. Your brain fog dissipates. You feel better.

> *Brandy: Age 49*
>
> *When I tell people about my journey to HRT I say, it's like driving the junkiest car you've ever owned: every check engine light is on and when you get up in the morning to start it it's like rah-rah-rah-rah-rah-rah. It's not that you don't have enough gasoline, it's not that the oil's bad, it's that your internal parts are not working anymore. They're just all misfiring and need to be tuned up.*

The first time I went to Cunningham Clinic, I'd just gotten off work. It was a very common thing for me to nod off, so I asked the receptionist to wake me up if I happened to fall asleep while I was waiting for my appointment. I was exhausted all the time.

True to form, I woke up to a tap on my shoulder when it was time for my appointment.

"Sorry if I was sleeping. I sleep a lot. I hope that you can fix that," I said. "Not a lot of stuff works for me."

"We will," was the answer.

One of the many reasons I fell asleep all the time was I wasn't sleeping well at night. I'd wake up at 1:00 or 2:00 in the morning, make a cup of tea and went back to bed an hour later. Four months after I began treatment, I began to sleep through the night and I wasn't so tired all day.

Next, my mental clarity began to return. I noticed a huge difference in sharpness, followed by improvements in my hair, dry skin, and my weight. I couldn't believe it, and neither could my husband who actually complained that we didn't cuddle as much because I wasn't freezing all the time!

When I went back and saw my regular doctor she asked, "How's the Wellbutrin treating you? Do you need anything different?"

"I weaned myself off." I'm a nurse so I know how to do that with caution. "Now that my hormones are balanced my depression is gone."

I'm sure she wasn't thrilled because my (then) doctor was against bioidentical hormones and supplements but was quick to put me on an antidepressant. I feel like that was a real injustice because she did so without looking at my hormones first.

All I needed was some simple blood work that needed to be evaluated.

For me, the improvement in my overall health was a big game changer. It changed my mental status. I felt whole. I wish I had done all of this sooner because I was dealing with so much— I was so overwhelmed taking care of a son who had intensive special needs and another who had a full, active life. I know for sure I would have been a better mother just because I was so run down all the time. I wouldn't have had to fake that I was happy and together and rested. I could have had more energy to face things that I was dealing with. I could have been able to see clearly the things I needed to eliminate in my life.

I'm so thankful now to feel so...how I should feel.

GETTING HORMONES INTO THE BODY

Hormones can be taken by pill, cream, injections, patch, troche, or pellets and there are different brands and compounds within each of these categories. In this chapter we will discuss the pros and cons of different types of medications and what I've found to be the most optimal ways to get the proper dosage into the body.

THYROID

Thyroid is always administered in pill form, but there are two different general types: synthetic or desiccated.

The American Thyroid Society has a position statement about why it's important to treat to the TSH and why Synthroid, or its generic levothyroxine (both of which are synthetic T4), should be the number one medication prescribed. They believe that because TSH level can be measured, it gives the practitioner the ability to monitor the client's levels to keep thyroid function within proper levels. As I've mentioned, it's not the TSH level that matters, but the Free T3 saturation rate and don't forget we need to check a Ferritin level to make sure the Free T3 can even get into the cell to work.. In other words, is the thyroid functional at the cellular level?

I prefer to prescribe what is known as a desiccated thyroid called Armour or NP Thyroid which is a combination of T3 and T4 at the ratio required at the cellular level to be functional. As a result, it doesn't matter if you make deiodinase or not, you get what you need at the cellular level in a pill.

99% of clients do better on desiccated thyroid, I always let people know it is a porcine product in case they have a religious restriction, are vegan, or have a food sensitivity.

When I prescribe a synthetic thyroid. I have my clients take a combination of Synthroid and what's called Cytomel, or liothyronine, which is synthetic T3. The only problem is the short half-life, so you have to take a Synthroid or levothyroxine in the morning with one or two Cytomel and then another one or two Cytomel pills mid-day. Instead of one pill, it's three or four a day which can get complicated to take daily.

ESTROGEN

Estrogen, which I only prescribe for women, is available as a cream, troche, pill, or in pellet form. Estrogen protects a woman against both heart disease and Alzheimer's, and is responsible for vaginal secretions, as well as skin and tissue integrity. We don't give a man estrogen, but they do have naturally occurring estrogen and we want that balance to continue along their hormone replacement therapy trajectory. For men receiving testosterone hormone replacement therapy, estrogen is typically 20 to 50. If a man's estrogen goes higher than that we worry about how much fat is in the body, and we might take a harder look at their body mass index and their fat ratios and make adjustments accordingly. If it goes lower than that we worry about osteoporosis and greater fracture risk. Men get their estrogen from aromatizing or converting testosterone over into estrogen so as their testosterone falls, so does their estrogen which can be a problem.

ESTROGEN IN PILL FORM

We have all taken pills and they would seem to be the simplest and safest way to get a needed substance into the body. However, this is not necessarily the case with hormones. For women, when estrogen is delivered via pill, the molecular structure of the estrogen is changed in the liver, which increases the risk of blood clot and strokes. It's the same reason that oral birth control pills (oral estrogen) have a warning on the label stating there is an increased risk of blood clot and/or strokes. As a result, I do not prescribe estrogen via a pill because I don't increase risks when there are other options. Bioidentical progesterone, on the other hand, which is taken with estrogen in peri and post-menopausal women (who still have a uterus), is well tolerated and safe in pill form.

TROCHE

A troche is a small dissolvable square that is placed between the cheek and teeth where it dissolves. It's very easy to dose, and it's very easy to take. Troches taste terrible, but that's certainly not a dealbreaker. My issues with troches are that they don't last long enough and they can atrophy the mouth over time. It's fine for people to use troches for six to twelve months. Six to twelve years is a different story. Because I play the long game and want what we're doing to be good for today and next week and next year, I prefer other methods of getting hormones into the system.

PATCHES AND CREAMS

Hormone patches and creams are a safe and potentially effective option, but the skin serves as a barrier to the body, so absorption can be an issue. Clients don't always get reliable, steady dosing because patches can have adhesion issues, sites must be rotated, and one area, like the right hip may absorb better than, say, the left outer thigh. The other issue with creams is they can be dangerous for little kids and animals. If you inadvertently rub against someone after applying the cream, you will dose that person. Estrogen cream can make a small dog produce milk. Testosterone cream will make that same small dog go bald. Creams can be bioactive for hours, and if you don't do a full scrub of your hands after application and open a door, it's on that door handle for whoever comes through behind you. Again, adults probably need a little, so that's not necessarily a problem, but small humans and animals can be very affected.

I actually had a client whose husband rubbed testosterone cream onto his pec at night, and she snuggled her cheek right next to his bare chest. She was 70 years old and had a hysterectomy with her ovaries removed, yet her testosterone level was perfect.

"Where are you getting it?" I asked her.

"I'm not getting any testosterone," she told me.

"But your labs are perfect."

In questioning her, we figured out that she had to be assimilating the testosterone through contact with her husband, but she didn't believe she was dosing through her face until he switched from creams to pellets.

"I can't function," she said, practically crawling into my office three weeks later.

Her labs showed that she had gone through a rapid testosterone withdrawal, and we started her on her own HRT plan.

For creams to work safely, the user has to put them on a patch of skin that is not touching somebody else, even during sexy time, and then cover that area with clothing.

One area of excellent absorption for creams is intravaginally because the skin is vascular, so you get a better uptake. However, it must be placed intravaginally after sex so that the client doesn't dose her partner.

I have some women who use an estrogen patch because they are perimenopausal, meaning they go in and out of menopause every other month. A patch is great because they can use it when they need it. If, all of the sudden, they have breast tenderness, they know they ovulated that month and might get a period. So, they can just rip off the patch, and it's gone in a day. A patch is a really convenient way to get women through perimenopause because they will literally ovulate one month, not for two months, ovulate for three months, and then not for four. In that situation, a patch for the estrogen part of that woman's HRT is going to be better than a cream.

I often use a vaginal cream in women who cannot have systemic estrogen. Since a transvaginal cream typically doesn't leave the vaginal vault, it is a great option to reach for in certain situations. Some women can't use systemic estrogen because they are currently receiving treatment for an estrogen-positive cancer, or have had breast, uterine, or ovarian cancer treatment. I also cannot give a woman systemic estrogen after the seventh decade of life in the complete absence of estrogen. One of the ways estrogen protects the brain is by regulating the tau protein. At some point in the seventh decade of a woman's life after menopause, or in the complete absence of estrogen for approximately 25 years, that tau protein can twist, and then I don't want to replicate it anymore because that could hasten the onset of dementia and other neurological diseases. In clients who start HRT more than 25 years after menopause—biologic or surgical—I'll go with testosterone therapy and vaginal estrogen.

We have a client in our practice who had a total hysterectomy with her ovaries removed when she was in her 50s and started HRT with my practice in her mid-80s. She came in three years ago leaning on a walker taking slow, shuffling, careful steps. After treating her with testosterone, she now walks independently and carries the walker. One day she came in for an appointment, put the walker down, and walked fluidly across the room to sit down.

"Kimberly, I've got a problem," she said.

"Yes, ma'am, how can I help you?" I asked.

"I have a boyfriend."

"That's great," I said.

"No." She pointed down at her lap. "It's like the Sahara."

Thank goodness we were still in masks, so she didn't see my smile. "I can fix that."

I gave her a prescription for vaginal estrogen cream, which she grasped from my hand. She then proceeded to grab her purse, slung it across her shoulder, picked up the walker she didn't need anymore because the testosterone has given her all this muscle tone, and started walking out the door. She stopped in the doorway and turned back to me. "Good, because I'm telling you, it's the desert down there."

And off she went.

A few months later, she reported that all was *very* well.

Vaginal estrogen, used twice a week, helps with tissue integrity. It also relieves the feeling of broken glass during or after intercourse, which is caused by the absence of estrogen in the vaginal vault. The estrogen also helps with the tissue integrity around the urethra and the chronic UTIs where the tissue is excoriated where the urine comes out. Vaginal estrogen helps a lot with improving sphincter tone, urinary continence, as well as vaginal vault tissue integrity and juiciness.

Vaginal estrogen is not going to protect the heart or the brain, but the testosterone will offer some protection against both heart disease and dementia. The vaginal estrogen helps with sexy time—but it's for after sex, not before, because if he gets trans-penis infusions of estrogen, he's going to get sore nipples, cry all the time, and he won't want to have sex.

TESTOSTERONE

As I've said, I strongly advocate for testosterone for both men and women. It is available as an injection, creams, troches, or pellet. Let's take a look at the various methods of assimilating this crucial hormone:

PILLS

Testosterone can't be taken orally because it is broken down by stomach acid. There are a few compounding pharmacies working on a special pill form of testosterone that is absorbed through the lymphatic channels in the small intestine, but we don't have good data yet showing absorption rates, so I'm avoiding testosterone pills for now.

PATCHES, GELS, AND CREAMS

I like patches, gels, and creams for testosterone but have the same reservations as I do with estrogen—namely issues with effective uptake through the skin and the risk to small children and pets. When women use estrogen or testosterone cream, they need to use it regularly. A lot of testosterone's benefits are in disease prevention, and so if a woman takes it just when she's feeling sluggish, she's not getting the steady-state dose protection that other modalities would give her.

INJECTIONS

Testosterone is the only hormone administered in injection form and typically prescribed just for men. Women don't usually utilize injections, but they can. The problem is the testosterone goes from zero to 3,000, back down to zero. Then, it's lather, rinse, and repeat regularly. Some doctors have gotten a little bit better by dividing the dose and giving it over two or three times in the week, but the client will start running out of intramuscular injection sites and has a higher risk of infection and nodule formation. If you are putting a needle into your quadriceps or into your glute three times a week, you're not going to have a healthy muscle in 20 years.

The other the problem is that a man who takes testosterone via injection will go from zero to super high repeatedly, and that can make the hair fall out and cause other side effects like facial or back acne, excessive sweating, and mood changes. We don't know why, but there is also an uptick in the risk of prostate cancer and prostate enlargement or hypertrophy that is exclusive to shots. It's not in the pellets or the creams. This may be caused by the solution which is emulsified using cottonseed, grapeseed, and even hemp oil, and clients report it to be a painful injection. There is nothing wrong with the actual testosterone, so the oil may be the culprit in both the burn felt during the injection and the irritation of the prostate. It also could be the bounce, but if the prostate is so big you've got to take Flomax or Avodart to try to shrink it and that medication causes erectile dysfunction which leads to taking ED medications, it feels medically like we're chasing our tails.

TROCHES

Troches are a viable option, but eventually lead to mouth issues as I mentioned, so I don't prescribe them for long term HRT.

PELLETS FOR ESTROGEN AND TESTOSTERONE

My personal preference, pure and simple, is for pellets—particularly to administer testosterone.

Pellets were developed in 1939 for women who had radical hysterectomies. I like pellets because they are easy to place, they provide steady dosing, and they don't have a lot of side effects or issues.

I would say 95% of my clients are on pellet therapy. They are just the easiest delivery method, the most economical, and they travel really well. It clears customs just fine and doesn't care what time zone you're in. I had a client who was going to a country where you couldn't take controlled substances, so we made sure he got his pellets before he went. He joked that I just made him into a mule—drugged with testosterone.

At Cunningham Clinic, we use clinical guidelines and use FDA approved clinical tools like a dosing site, which has been validated by studies of over 60,000 men and 60,000 women who were followed for many years.

Based on the client's height, weight, lab values, and medical history, we decide on the ideal dose. We always err on the side of caution as part of my *start low and go slow* approach to health care.

So, if we're going with estrogen in a perimenopausal woman, obviously, we don't want to give her a full dose of estrogen, because on the months she ovulates, she's going to go too high. When estrogen is too high, she can't wear a bra because her breasts are too sore. So, to be careful with that, we would just give her a partial dose.

We always start off conservatively, and then bring the client back in after four or six weeks to check labs. Some people run a little higher, some people run a little lower based on individual response rates.

The most important aspect is the answer to the question, "How are you feeling?"

Post-pellet goal ranges are based on really good data, but where the person falls best within that range is an individual, customized plan that is based on the answer to that all-important question. We figure out where the sweet spot is for that individual client, and it can take a couple of rounds of pellets to sort that out.

Here's where it gets really interesting. When you're younger and your ovaries or testes are functioning, you have both a baseline steady state of hormone as well as a spike right after something taxing like running a race, hiking up the side of a mountain, or navigating something stressful. That's because ovaries and testes are solid organs that produce hormones. What that means is blood flows past the solid organ, picks up hormones and delivers them downstream to where you need it. Pellets are the only form of HRT that offer endocrine mimicry – copying exactly what the body was able to do when it was functional. This is why, once we start HRT, all hormone blood testing needs to be hormones at rest, as in no exercise the morning of the blood draw. I had a patient once ask me if I had just given her a new ovary with her pellets. "Functionally, I sure did," was my reply. I will always reach for the most natural, bioidentical, human identical option for health and wellness. Pellets fit that perfectly.

BIOTE® PELLETS

There are a lot of pellet companies, cream companies, and compounding pharmacies out there. When I started my practice, there were four. Now, less than a decade later, there are nearly 100 companies in the bioidentical hormone replacement therapy realm. New companies pop up regularly because this is what women and men want, because this is what is working.

Some companies offer cheaper products and make various claims, but I use Biote® pellets which are produced by a 503B certified compounding pharmacy. Biote's® testosterone and estrogen are derived from Central American yams, which contain hormones that are identical to humans. I love that this product is sustainable, bioidentical, effective and, best of all, doesn't include harming horses in the manufacturing process. They are not only the safest, and most reliable, but come in all different milligrams, so I can customize the dose. In addition, Biote® guarantees a maximum 3% milligram swing, batch to batch, and only 3% deviation of performance batch to batch. I have great faith in the product and the company as they do extensive research and publication of their findings on bioidentical hormone replacement therapy, safety, and efficacy. In addition, they're currently the only ones in the country that I see doing continuing education.

You cannot get a patent for bioidentical estrogen or testosterone because they exist in nature. Currently the FDA doesn't allow you to submit something for approval without a patent so it's quite the catch-22. Especially when doctors say they won't write for something that's not FDA approved. What is FDA approved is the manufacturing process to make the pellets, and the Biote® dosing algorithms which utilize multiple lab values and client history parameters to recommend starting doses which we utilize rigorously.

PELLET INSERTION

Pellet insertion is an easy, straightforward procedure. The client lies on their side, and I expose the hip or the flank. I put a little sterile drape around the area, clean the skin, give a little numbing shot, and make a tiny incision. The pellets go in with something called a trocar, which is like a surgical steel straw with a plunger.

And then it's just three little steri-strips and a bandage.

I teach pellet insertion certification for Biote®. In my classes, I always tell the providers that, for female clients, *if it's not in the thong it's wrong* because a woman should be able to rock a thong on the beach, and nobody should know she gets pellet therapy but her. We always keep the incision where it can be hidden. Most men have hair on their butt, so you're not going to see it, no matter what. It's already camouflaged.

I instruct my female clients that there is no soaking or exercising for three days. They can have a shower but no pool, bathtub, hot tub, lake, or ocean because I don't want the incision to get infected. And no exercising the lower body for three days because I don't want that glute to flex and possibly work the pellets back out.

One of my clients called me the evening after her procedure and asked, "Am I allowed to have sex?"

"Yes," I said, "Have as much sex as you like, but you're not allowed to flex your glute."

My client started listing off various positions.

"Just don't flex your butt," I said.

The reason I give my clients this warning is that when you flex that butt muscle, it compresses the subcutaneous fat. The pellets sit (painlessly) in the fat, and you could push the pellet up through the fat globules to the skin. If the skin gets hold of it, the pellet might extrude (pop back out through the original insertion point) in three to six weeks.

I tell women it's like their nails, it's dry but not set, for three days. For the men, I say it's like the paint on the wall. It's dry but not set—you can't hang the pictures on it yet. You can't flex yet. For men, it's five to seven days without exercise if they are getting the smaller pellets and seven days if they're getting the larger pellets. And no soaking for the five to seven days, just like the women, to reduce the risk of infection.

When clients complain, and it's rarely about any pain or the incision, it's that they can't exercise for a few days after. I tell them, you can stroll and you can walk the dog, but you just can't run, bike, power walk, or do leg-day workouts. I tell the ladies, "I get nine days a year and you get the rest in a functioning body." For the men, I tell them, "I get them 15 days a year, and they get the rest of the year to feel great."

HORMONE REPLACEMENT METHODS

Synthetic:
- Pills
- Patches
- Shots

Bioidentical:
- Pills
- Patches
- Creams/Gels
- Pellets

Potential & Unnecessary Effects of Oral Estrogen Therapy:
- Breast tenderness
- Increased risk of endometrial cancer & breast cancer
- Weight gain
- Vaginal bleeding
- Headaches
- Nausea & vomiting
- Fluid retention
- Blood clots
- Leg cramps

Patches:
- Estradiol levels better than pills, but not as good as pellets
- Adhesive problem
- Need to be changed throughout the week
- Some weight gain, but less fluid retention than being on synthetic or horse estrogen
- *45% of people do not absorb hormones through the skin!*

Creams/Gels:
- Did you apply enough?
- Rub it in 1-2 times daily—A PAIN!
- Short half-life
- Is it even absorbing?
- Can transfer to others (babies/pets)
- Most important estriol (as in the product BiEst) DOES NOT protect the bones, muscles, and libido

Injectable Testosterone:
- Uneven absorption
- Significant "roller coaster" effect
- 99% synthetic hormone
- Significant adverse effects:
    - ◊ Liver toxicity, heart disease
    - ◊ Elevates LDL, VLDL, Decreases HDL Cholesterol
- ALWAYS wears off before time for next shot . . . *Makes Guys Really CRANKY!*

Bio-identical Hormone Pellets:
- Natural, plant-derived compounds
- Same molecular structure as human hormones
- Lasts longer than other treatments, up to 4-6 months
- Most widely studied form of natural hormone replacement therapy
- Provides steady stream of hormone in your blood
- Individualized dosing
- Injected under the skin
- Only option that offers endocrine mimicry
- DON'T EVEN KNOW IT'S THERE!

What is Biote® Therapy?
Helps Body Return to Normal Hormonal Balance & Physiological State
- Right kind of hormone *(Bio-Identical)*
- Right amounts *(Individualized Dosing)*
- Right delivery system *(Pellets)*
- Safe: hundreds of studies, 75 yrs experience, used in 5 continents
- Clinically Effective: even levels—*"NO Roller Coaster Effect"*
- Convenience/Compliance: Implanted a few times a year
- Low side-effect profile
- *BEST* method to increase bone density
- No evidence of increased breast cancer risk - does not stimulate breast tissue
- No increase in blood clots, heart attack or stroke
- Protective to the *breast, bones, brains, heart, & relationships*

SIDE EFFECTS

When a woman reports to me that she is experiencing hot flashes and vaginal dryness (and all of her risk factors check out) I prescribe estrogen and progesterone. Too much estrogen in a post-menopausal woman can cause breast tenderness—and if she still has a uterus—temporary bleeding or spotting. When that happens, we fine-tune to make sure she is balanced and those symptoms resolve. I make sure to dose conservatively in order to get her in the post-pellet estrogen range of 20 to 60 and improvement of low estrogen symptoms.

As I mentioned in a previous chapter, the 2003 Women's Health Initiative study was stopped due to the risk of breast cancer. In the aftermath, all but one of those researchers recanted and said it was never the estrogen. If a woman has an estrogen positive cancer in her body however, estrogen could feed it and it might grow a bit faster. That is a scary sentence, but it's actually a good thing if the cancer is in the uterus. Endometrial lining cancers are silent cancers. I've found endometrial cancer six times now in my years of providing HRT. The estrogen didn't cause the cancer, but it did cause the cancer to show itself. All of those women had to undergo a hysterectomy, but none had any spread beyond the uterus. Because estrogen made them bleed, we were able to find the cancer in a timeline that saved their lives.

WOMEN'S HEALTH INITIATIVE TRIAL . . . A FLAWED STUDY!

- 41% Increase in stroke (Wrong route – never take estrogen as a pill)
- 26% Increase in breast cancer (ONLY in the synthetic progesterone arm of the study)
- Twice the rate of blood clots (Again, don't take estrogen as a pill)

This was a FLAWED study! After this trial many women were left with NO alternative for hormone balance and symptom relief.

Sadly, there have been safe, alternative methods available for years. The message should have been, "Let's take a closer look at hormones . . ."

VITAMIN D

It is important to stay at a Vitamin D level of 70-100. Above 100, bone reabsorption is possible and at very high levels nausea, vomiting, confusion, and medical conditions like hypercalcemia or kidney issues are possible. Vitamin D is fat soluble, so you can store it up, which is a good thing, but regular blood tests to make sure you don't overshoot the mark are important. We check Vitamin D levels every six to 12 months to make sure we are in that optimal range.

B VITAMINS

B vitamins are water soluble, so if you have good kidney function, you just flush them out of your system. You can get temporary headaches, a metal taste on your tongue, numbness in your hands, and tingling. But, again, it's short-lived and resolves. These side effects typically occur in people who take more than the recommended dose or have an appropriate B_{12} level and then go with their friends to an IV bar and get talked into a B_{12} shot they don't need.

THYROID MEDICATION

Over-replacement of thyroid can cause diarrhea and/or rapid heart rate. In those over the age of 75, too much thyroid medication can cause atrial fibrillation (an abnormal heart rhythm). Regular lab draws every three to six months when getting started are part of a good thyroid plan.

TESTOSTERONE AND MEN

A high testosterone level in men is typically not a problem in the short term. In men who do testosterone shots, it's not uncommon for them to hit as high as 2,000 to 3,000 on a blood draw within an hour after the injection. High levels of testosterone can cause an increase in hemoglobin and hematocrit, which is the thickness, if you will, of your blood. There's no data showing that testosterone therapy increases the risk of blood clot in men or women, but in general, we don't want a hemoglobin and hematocrit that's climbing, so we watch for that.

We want to keep men below 1,450 on a sustained level because a supraphysiologic (very high) testosterone level over for six months can down-regulate sex drive in a man. They might build enormous muscle, but when the testosterone goes that high, the hair thins and the testicles will shrink. The only way to re-up those receptor sites is to keep the testosterone at 800 or less for a year.

We're not doing any of this to impact sexy time for the worse!

In my clinic, the goal is up to 1,100 for most men post-pellet, at the 8 week post pellet lab test. That way, I know it's going to last for four or five months depending on the size of the pellets we're using. We know that elite male athletes naturally have higher testosterone, so I'll run them a little bit higher. I have clients who've played for professional sports teams or are retired MMA fighters. For those men to feel normal, they really need to be up to 1,400. I will also, occasionally, treat men with chronic pain, autoimmune conditions that are not well controlled, or certain medical conditions to a higher testosterone goal, but I will get them up there slowly, just making sure the other labs stay stable.

Along with the down-regulation of sex drive, the second thing that can happen with men is called aromatization. That is where some men process their testosterone in a way that causes it to tumble over into estrogen. High estrogen in men causes sore nipples, moodiness, and they can cry easily. The higher the testosterone the higher, of course, the risk, because there's a bigger base to tumble over into a bigger amount of estrogen. Men who have a lot of adipose tissue, which is fat, need to be run a little bit lower because that fat's already making some estrogen. If a man does aromatize, and some men just do, I can put him on a medication to block that process.

The last thing I screen for is testicular shrinkage, scrotal retraction, or both as a result of testosterone therapy. It is an uncommon side effect when the testosterone is regulated properly, occurring in only two percent or less of men, but it can happen. Of the 900 plus clients in my practice, four men have had testicular shrinkage. However, because the functional part of their sexual abilities returned, only one client had any interest in being treated for what was a small change in their testicular/scrotal size, and only then because he and his partner were in an open relationship and were concerned about appearance. There are medications I can put men on to restore their physical appearance if necessary.

TESTOSTERONE AND WOMEN

With testosterone therapy, women typically feel the best at a post-pellet level of 125 to 250. That is the level at which we know it's typically going to last for four months.

Within the normal range, we go by two things. *How are you feeling? Do you have any side effects?* If someone comes in at 150, and they don't feel better, I can go up. If they come in at 200 and feel like a rock star, but they're having some side effects, clearly, I can take them back down a little bit with their next round of hormone replacement therapy.

Side effects from too much testosterone include an increase in facial hair, acne, an increase in sweating at the top end, and, very rarely, hair thinning. For a woman, that would typically be at the temples.

Interestingly enough, facial hair is a sign that a female needs testosterone. Everyone has a mom or an aunt or a grandma with a full mustache and maybe even a little soul patch and they're probably not on hormone replacement therapy! What testosterone will do is make hair grow thicker, faster, stronger, longer—including any chin hairs. Sometimes it's just a matter of that hair growing in faster, and so it seems like it's more, but it's that same hair coming in a few days sooner.

Thinning hair at the temples resolves when the testosterone comes back down. The acne, if it happens, typically occurs at the beginning of hormone replacement therapy. It helps to think of hormone replacement therapy like puberty. Puberty is the body's transition from non-functioning hormones to functioning hormones. That's exactly what we're doing, only we can get there in six weeks instead of six years.

STACKING

I'm really careful about when we plan for re-pelleting women due to what is called stacking. Stacking is where that last dose hasn't completely waned, so I always get blood levels when the woman comes in more frequently than three months to make sure the peak doesn't go too high. Any time a woman stacks, she can get a breakout, three or four extra chin hairs, and her hair could thin. That's why I get lots of labs, and we make sure they're in the correct range. Any time we change the dose or the timeline, we get more labs.

CLITORAL ENLARGEMENT

Clitoral enlargement is a very rare side effect. Mild to moderate clitoral enlargement is typically the clitoris returning back to its normal presentation.

Sometimes, I'll get a call from someone who says, "I'm growing a penis."

They aren't.

And when they come in, they have a very normal presentation. True clitoral enlargement is rare and usually improves by simply lowering the testosterone dose for the next round of pellets.

MALE BIRTH CONTROL

Any form of testosterone—cream, injection, troche, or pellet—can reduce the total number of sperm. For pellet therapy, that sperm count reduction lasts about six to eight months, depending on the size of the pellets used but any form of testosterone can cause permanent sperm reduction. We always check to make sure our male clients have completed their families and are not trying to conceive. We also counsel our male pellet recipients that testosterone is not complete male birth control, and that they should use additional birth control. In females, testosterone often increases fertility as the body gets stronger and libido returns, increasing the activity required for conception.

PELLET EXTRUSION

One side effect unique to pellets is the possibility of extrusion. When a pellet extrudes, it typically happens a few weeks after insertion. The pellet will come back out of the little, tiny line where the incision was. It looks like a little spider bite or bug bite, and I can push on it, and there's a little bit of fluid. Sometimes, I can see the pellet. I touch it with a scalpel and pop it right out.

In women, it's always the big pellet—100 milligrams of testosterone they needed is now gone. When this happens, I just go an inch and a half or two inches further away and insert a new pellet and give them a boost. I don't charge for the boost, but they are resetting the clock for three days of no soaking or exercising. Thankfully, it doesn't happen very often.

SCARRING

Most people heal from the pellet insertions with no sign of any incision. Those prone to scarring may have little white lines at pellet insertion spots, but they're tiny and you have to get very close to see them.

SLOW AND STEADY

It is very easy to avoid the side effects mentioned above with conservative dosing. There are people who walk in the door desperate for anything to get them feeling better and they're like, "Give me all of it today. I have to have it."

I had a woman come in thinking the pellets were inserted anally and she was totally okay with that. When I explained that an anal hormone suppository wasn't a thing and that I was going to place the pellets under the skin in the hip area she said, "You can put them anywhere you want. I'm desperate."

I can usually talk some sense into clients by promising to get them there safely. What I don't want to do is take them from this place of desperation and then throw a bunch of side effects on top of it in two weeks when they're not even better yet.

There is one very small, typically unavoidable side effect, for men and women the first time they get their pellets—crankiness. I tell everyone to prepare to be an unreasonable teenager for one to two days sometime in the first three weeks after the first round of pellets. I can't predict which day—but that they need to give everyone around them a pass that first month on HRT. It's not the time to let the complete stranger who parked their car over the line know what you think of them!

DON'T STOP

There are a host of medicines that, once started, are necessary forever. If you need to start taking thyroid medication, that's what you're probably going to take, adjusting the dosage as necessary, for the remainder of your life. The same holds true for hormone replacement therapy.

If clients stop their hormone replacement therapy, they will age quickly. I am able to give them back ten or 20 years, but underneath they are getting older and the natural ability to do the processes we've replaced is waning. They are not going to go back to where they were ten years ago, but wherever they were going to age to today. That's a long way to fall, so people typically don't quit. Besides, they feel amazing, and they want to be in a body that functions. If (and when) they restart, the gap they aged doesn't always come back. There's a new baseline.

Estrogen and testosterone reduce the risk of Alzheimer's in women. Testosterone reduces the risk of Alzheimer's in men. In men and women, testosterone provides core stability. Older people can actually put their pants on, lift their legs, and put on their shoes. When

I was in geriatrics, these were the measures by which people would fail and be required to go into some sort of assisted or long-term care.

My oldest Cunningham Clinic client was 92 when she moved to California a few years ago to help out her son whose general health was worse than hers. She's still spry, healthy, and hoping she can convince him to get on hormones, so he can feel as good as she does!

Now, my oldest client is a ruddy, healthy 87.

I have a client who goes to the same family practice doctor every year. And every year his doctor says, "You can't do that testosterone. It's bad for you."

And yet, every year, his labs are perfect, his body fat percentage is perfect, and the only medication he takes is a low dose thyroid pill. Meanwhile, my client tells me his doctor has lost most of his hair. The doctor's shoulders used to be square. Now, they're sloped. He's got a potbelly and looks kind of grayish. Every year, my client says to his doctor, "You know, you should go over to my HRT clinic and have them check your blood."

"I don't believe in that," the doctor says.

They look 20 years apart, but they're the same age—the same phenomenon I've been watching over the better part of the last decade.

POTENTIAL TEMPORARY CONCERNS OF PELLET INSERTIONS (usually just the first round of pellets)

- Fluid retention
  - ◊ Occasionally occurs with the first insertion, and especially when done in hot, humid weather conditions
- Swelling of the hands & feet
  - ◊ Common in hot, humid weather conditions
  - ◊ Less then 2% of clients experience any side effect
- Breast tenderness & nipple sensitivity
- Uterine spotting or bleeding in women receiving estrogen
- Mood swings & irritability
- Pellet extrusion
- Facial breakout
- Reduction in testicular size
- Reduction in sperm count

A YEAR IN THE LIFE

At Cunningham Clinic, the journey to better health starts with that initial lab draw. It doesn't take long to do that all important blood draw, but there is a comprehensive questionnaire to fill out and go through. We want a health history complete with height, weight, medications, supplements, surgeries, medical diagnoses, and all the doctors someone has seen or is seeing.

For men, I have specific questions about birth control because testosterone tends to suppress sperm production, and I want to make sure my client is not actively trying to have another child. In woman we don't give testosterone in the third trimester, but I've helped quite a few clients get pregnant. Again, we always talk about what their plans are and what they are using for birth control. I need to know if the client is going to have surgery soon. If so, we want to get some testosterone on board before a trip to the operating room to help faster, better healing.

One week after the blood draw, clients come back in for the results. We go over everything in person and what I recommend in light of what we see. If I believe pellets are the way to go and the client is ready, we'll start them on their path that day.

Eight weeks later, I have the client back in. That's where we have the follow-up questions:

How are you doing?

How are you feeling?

Do you notice a difference yet?

We order another blood draw to check the numbers. If we feel it's necessary, I will do a boost—another little procedure with some more pellets, a little bit more estrogen, estrogen and testosterone, or just testosterone. That boost should get the client to therapeutic doses, both to match the therapeutic range we're shooting for, as well as for symptom improvement.

From that point on, I see the client on average once every four months. I have some men that come in at five months because they're getting the large pellets, and I have some women who need to come back every three months because they're marathon runners or smokers. People will use up the pellets in direct correlation to cardiac output so my couch potatoes can go longer than my workout instructors. Any time I change the dose, I'm going to get another set of labs in four or eight weeks.

Once a year, I do my big annual panel, and I always get that as a trough level two weeks before they are due to come in for their next round of pellets to ensure their timeline is correct and they are not at risk of stacking their hormones. There are other things that can influence whether or not the hormones are working, and so there might be a need for some other labs from time to time.

Often, people will come in for their initial visit with a laundry list of maladies they want me to fix. Even though they may have important issues that need to be addressed, my priority is to get the hormones fixed. I'm not saying that gastroesophageal reflux isn't important. Chronic constipation is certainly important. And chronic joint pain first thing in the morning is definitely a problem. We will circle back to all these other maladies in about four months, and we're going to see what's left, and then we can chase those. Nine times out of ten, I ask a client about their list when they come in for their four-month visit and they're like, "My what? Oh, yeah, I don't even have that anymore."

We've worked to put back all the things that are missing in your body. We give you back your vitamins, your hormones, and your thyroid functionality. We give you back all the things you need to have a body that works—especially that long, lost healthy sex drive. The foundation for good health is, once again, solid.

I have two clients who divorced each other nearly 15 years ago. They are both seeing me for hormone replacement therapy and bad thyroids (which went bad on both of them 15 years ago) but here's where this gets interesting: *they each don't know the other is seeing me for hormone replacement therapy and healthy aging support.*

Both of them have independently said they keep bumping into each other and talk about each other as the love of their life. They both had four independent risk factors for depression that I've corrected with thyroid medication, B_{12}, Vitamin D, testosterone and/or testosterone and estrogen.

Is it any wonder that with fixed hormones and their depression in check they are in the process of getting back together?

Maureen: Age 62

Women born in the 1960s don't typically talk about what's going on during and after menopause. My mom didn't talk to me about it and I didn't know how to feel when I went through it. All I can say is that it isn't what I expected.

Once it ended, I just felt tired all the time, my skin was crepe-y under my arms and on my legs and I was itchy, dry, and flaky. Sex was painful for the first time in my life.

All my doctor said was, "You're getting older. What do you expect?"

I did have an expectation—to be able to live feeling healthy and active and not tired in my 60s and 70s. I wanted to enjoy the things I used to enjoy, but things were just dwindling. I was really bummed out. I was like, is this all there is?

Then, I found Cunningham Clinic. I had the bloodwork I needed and learned that everything was low— my estrogen, my testosterone, all my vitamins, and my thyroid. I had been wondering and asking about my thyroid for years, but it was just outside of the normal range, so my primary care doctor didn't feel the need to treat for it.

I started HRT. It took about eight months and a couple of visits to get things stabilized and I stopped waking up in the middle of the night and being unable to go back to sleep. I wasn't tired in the afternoons. My blood pressure, which was always slightly elevated, went back to normal. And my sex life improved because it was no longer painful. I'm a runner and I run four days a week. I used to be really, really achy and sore when I would get up in the morning and I don't feel any of that anymore. In fact, I feel better than I did in my 30's.

I can talk about HRT with conviction because it actually worked for me, and it is still working for me. I tell everyone because I want them to feel as good as I feel.

Lucy age 73

I think I look younger than I did before I started it and I seem to have more stamina than friends my age. I actually lost about five or six pounds immediately without doing anything. When I look in the mirror I don't look like I'm in my 40s, but I also don't look like I'm in my 70s.

Pellet therapy is very easy. Sometimes it stings a bit, but that's just a minor inconvenience. When I can't get to Cunningham Clinic I have a local provider in Florida where I live part of the year. I can tell if I've gone too long between pellets, so I'm not going to skip it. My energy kind of bottoms out and I don't care for that. I don't want to let aging take me down the tubes and I want to do as much as I can for as long as I can.

And this actually makes me feel good.

> **Melinda: Age 60**
>
> *Right after getting pellets there is that surge point. I enjoy it, because I feel like a 19-year-old and I'm acting like an 18-year-old. My husband definitely enjoys that part, too. I'm interested and initiate sex. The fact that hormones allow me to show my partner I'm interested is a huge deal emotionally for our marriage.*
>
> *When my pellets start to run low, my appointment at Cunningham Clinic is a priority.*
>
> *He'll say, "We've got to get you your pellets!"*

THE HORMONES ARE FIXED, BUT . . .

I have sexual wellness clients who come in having tried a variety of treatments that didn't work. It's not a surprise. Again, it's because testosterone is muscle tone, tissue integrity, blood vessel health and nerve endings. Unless there is testosterone, and hopefully estrogen (if that's safe to do) on board, the other treatments are less effective. Fixing the hormones comes first. We don't jump into anything else because actually a lot of the times, no further intervention is necessary. After bioidentical hormone replacement therapy, clients are often good to go.

About ten percent of the time however, hormone replacement therapy is not enough. Women don't quite get enough vaginal tone or clitoral stimulus back. Depending on how long a woman's been without her hormones, and how much damage she sustained in childbirth—big baby, little pelvis—sometimes there's additional repair work to be done. Thankfully, there are a number of effective, medically proven interventions that work well.

> **Andrea Age 51**
>
> *I am not experiencing the high highs that people get from hormone replacement therapy in their sex life. The orgasms are not super intense. I don't know if that's hormones or my body, but I definitely know that I had zero interest in sex previously and now I have an interest. But the physical part of it, I haven't seen a huge difference in that. Not yet.*

SURGICAL LABIAPLASTY/VAGINOPLASTY—NOT MY FAVORITE SOLUTION

An overstretched labia is kind of like an earlobe—it's not going back without some sort of intervention. It's a problem when you ride a bike, when you have sex, and even when you wear the wrong underwear.

Labiaplasty is a surgical resection—a cutting and putting back together—to correct an overstretched labia. Similarly, Vaginoplasty involves going in, cutting the vaginal wall, pulling everything tighter circumferentially, and sewing it back up.

These procedures are difficult for a variety of reasons. All surgery involves risk—the risk of undergoing a surgical procedure, complications from anesthesia, and six to eight weeks of recovery that includes extensive discharge, blood, and potential infection. Clients have to cycle on and off antibiotics during this time, and it's hard to walk. And that is assuming all goes well. The bladder and urethra are right there, and the bowel is on the other side. Any time you go in and start cutting and sewing back together, things can go wrong. And do.

Surgical labiaplasty and vaginoplasty used to be the only truly viable options to have the vaginal vault tightened or the labia lifted. And while these procedures are still available, they are becoming increasingly obsolete due to effective non-surgical, in-office technologies like Morpheus V®, V-Tone®, Aviva®, and other devices that have been developed and are being utilized by gynecologists, urologists, and health practitioners for vaginal vault tightening and tissue integrity improvement. There have been a flood of new devices over the past ten years as nonsurgical options have come on the market, some of which have proved to work very well.

Let's take a look at some of these technologies:

MORPHEUS V®

The Morpheus V® is part of a device called the EmpowerRF™ platform which includes multiple handpieces that can be used to correct age and birth-trauma-related changes to the vagina, labia, and clitoris. It is used by gynecologists to do nonsurgical labia and vaginoplasties.

Initially developed as a radiofrequency micro-needling device for use on the face, neck, and body, the company developed a vaginal wand which utilizes both the radiofrequency and micro needling technique within the vaginal vault. As a result of using the Morpheus V®, there is tissue regeneration and vaginal tissue thickening in just three to four treatments, which are administered a month apart.

I do not currently offer this procedure in office but give referrals to various gynecological surgeons who do. My clients rave about the results.

> **Wendy: Age 60**
>
> *You drive yourself there, they numb you and give you a bit of nitrous and they do the Morpheus V procedure. It takes roughly two hours the first time but less the next time because each treatment works so well. You really can't Kegel or lubricate your way into the kind of results I noticed right away. I feel like I did down there long before menopause.*

VTONE®

VTone® also part of the EmpowerRF™ platform, is an FDA cleared technology which provides intravaginal electrical muscle stimulation and neuromuscular assistance to weak pelvic floor muscles. In essence, the VTone®, once inserted into the vagina, compels your muscles to kegel. You sit for 20 or 30 minutes for three sessions with your feet up in stirrups while the machine does the work for you. It's a little awkward, but it's not uncomfortable. As a result, after as few as three visits, you get muscular improvement, improved vaginal thickness, and relief from urinary incontinence.

AVIVA®

The Aviva®, part of the EmpowerRF™ platform, is a small non-surgical wand which is inserted inside the labia. The wand communicates with a receptor outside the labia using radiofrequency and heats the tissue up enough to tighten the fibroceptal network within the skin. It's a 15 minute procedure which helps a lax, long labia tighten back up. There can be some bleeding, swelling, and tenderness. But, unlike surgery, you can drive yourself home.

Once healed, the Aviva® treatment allows women to get out the Kama Sutra book and see if they can pretzel twist into something fun! In other words, they look and feel like their old sexy selves.

> *Lynne: Age 52*
>
> *Over the last four or five years I noticed some labial laxity even though I've never had children. HRT didn't quite do enough, so I decided to try out Aviva non-surgical vaginoplasty. I've done the first of three in office treatments. I was fully numbed and the recovery was very minor. I even drove myself home. There was one day where it felt like there was a baseball between my legs and I couldn't cross my legs for a week, but I was back to my life the next day.*
>
> *I've already noticed a real difference in the appearance of my labia. I kind of described them as looking like elephant ears before, but now everything is nice and tight and closer to my body. I just feel more confident about the way I look.*
>
> *I'm actually looking forward to my next treatment.*

EMSELLA™ CHAIR

EMSELLA™ is a completely non-invasive treatment to improve pelvic floor muscles. It utilizes electromagnetic energy to deliver thousands of pelvic floor muscle contractions in a single session. These contractions re-educate the muscles of incontinent patients and clinical studies showed up to 75% reduction in the use of urinary incontinence pads and a satisfaction rate after a series of three to five treatments. The EMSELLA™ is probably the easiest of the treatments as it is literally sitting in a special chair for thirty minutes – no need to even disrobe/get undressed. While it won't improve labial laxity or vaginal tissue quality, the bladder and pelvic floor improvements are impressive.

PRP SHOTS

Platelet Rich Plasma or PRP Shots for vaginal rejuvenation (also known as the O-shot™, the WoW™ shot and G-Shot™) are a game changer.

PRP injections started as treatments in orthopedic clinics to improve and treat sports-related injuries in the knees and elbows. Doctors then realized it could be used to great effect on other parts of the body including the penis and clitoris for improved blood flow and function. PRP injection treatment is relatively simple, very effective, and we offer it in the office.

For women, we put topical numbing all over the labia, into the vaginal vault, and onto the clitoris. We draw the blood and spin it down until we have 10 CCs of platelet-rich plasma. While PRP is often done with a regular blood tube centrifuge, we utilize a machine called the Magellan™, which separates the blood in exactly the specific gravity needed to administer this procedure.

At this point, the numbing cream has taken effect, so the woman feels little to no discomfort as we inject different points to improve sexual function. The first injection is just to the right and left of the vaginal opening and stimulates the stretch receptors on the legs of the clitoris. We then inject just underneath the urethra to improve sphincter tone and stimulate the G-spot or deep vaginal clitoral stimulus. Studies show that the injection point under the urethra can result in up to an 80% improvement of sphincter tone along the whole length of the urethra. The final location gets both the heart of the clitoris as well as the outermost part of the clitoris (where everybody puts the vibrator).

This injection series for women places the PRP strategically in all major parts of the clitoris and is like a wake-up. It's actually an irritant—a prescribed injury to get a specific response and repair. The goal is to get the little legs that go around the vaginal opening to wake up. We are also trying to get the G-spot or deep penetration to wake up. We want the entire clitoris to have feeling; we want the nerves and blood vessels to have erectile functionality.

After a PRP shot, nothing is to be inserted into the vagina for 24 hours. I warn clients they might feel like they rode a horse or a bike all day, so to expect to be tender that night and the next day.

It's a great procedure and appropriate clients who just need a little more oomph have it done every other year on average. It's kind of like Botox®, it will wear off, but it lasts a good 18 to 24 months.

Recently, two long-time clients who both got PRP shots (and are good friends) were in the clinic lobby.

One was doing jumping jacks shouting, "Look! No pee!"

"I didn't have that problem," her friend said. "But let me tell you about my sexy time!"

> ***Brandy: Age 49***
>
> *My sex drive has always been great—the sensation and feeling down there—but peeing my pants has been an ongoing problem even after HRT. I'm only 49, and I wouldn't have thought I'd have such problems with my bladder, but the last five years have been just terrible.*
>
> *I mentioned I was sick and tired of peeing my pants during one of my consultations and learned the PRP shot could be tailored for urinary incontinence and to improve my sphincter tone by as much as 80%.*
>
> *I had the treatment in July and took the grandkids to an indoor trampoline place they love in October. Once, before my treatment, I tried to jump and peed the pad I had to wear immediately. This time, I decided to try the trampoline again. I jumped on every one the place had and didn't have any issues at all! Recently, I went sledding. It was pretty steep and the drop usually makes me have to pee. Not this time.*
>
> *I would have been happy with any improvement, but I'm thrilled to say I'm at 100%. I'm getting really used to being dry!*

PELVIC FLOOR PT

If women are still having painful sex after the hormones are fixed, the vagina could be clamped down too tight or certain muscles might be misfiring. When it's clear this is the situation, I refer out to pelvic floor physical therapy. Some women have pain post-delivery or peri- and post-menopause as a result of spasm in the obturator and other pelvic floor muscles. There are many muscles which intertwine, and they do lots of different things. Transvaginal physical therapy is a specific specialty which is typically covered by insurance, and helps with muscle tone, innervation, and making sure all the muscles are firing correctly.

When these muscles are misfiring, you get to be really good friends with your pelvic floor physical therapist. Like me, they don't care about modesty and aren't squeamish in the slightest. They want you to have a functioning body. To that end, a well-trained, professional PT will always ask for and wait until you give consent for any treatment that involves internal vaginal or rectal work. An intimate treatment is something you will likely work up to as treatment plans include non-internal work as well.

Years ago, I had a patient come in for a lab panel after having her second child. She was recovering from her pregnancy well and already back to running, but sex was just too painful, and she was getting frustrated. Her labs all looked great, so I referred her to an amazing pelvic floor physical therapist for a series of pelvic floor PT sessions. Within two months, all of the muscles in her pelvic floor were working together and firing correctly, and she and her husband were very satisfied with the results. It was about ten years later that I started the same couple on hormone replacement therapy, and they are still competing in 10k races together.

DELICATE SUBJECTS

For someone who has a history of sexual assault or any kind of assault, treatments like an O-Shot™ can be traumatic. Even though the client is numb, you're putting a needle into the vaginal vault.

To allay any panic response, we make sure to prop a client's head up instead of laying them all the way flat. Because we ask questions about history of sexual trauma, we get answers that help us to help our clients feel more comfortable.

I also have women who come in and say, "I haven't had an orgasm in a year."

"Is that with somebody else or by yourself?" I ask.

When they say, "I can get there by myself, but I don't like my husband anymore," we have a whole different set of circumstances to work through.

I can tell you that to like somebody else you have to like yourself first. When you don't like yourself, you certainly can't like anybody else. I believe what I do is fix people's ability to appreciate living in a body that functions, which allows them to start to like themselves, and that translates into liking somebody else. Even their spouses!

Just like you can't build muscle without testosterone, whatever you're doing in therapy, meditation, or for self-help isn't going to work until we support the rest of you. Why? Because there's too much noise; too much in the way.

I have found that when it comes to sexual dysfunction, women are usually in their heads and men are in their penis. Sexual dysfunction can be a physiological or a psychological problem. Nine times out of ten, if I fix the physiological or the measurable diagnostic problem, the psychological ones become much less severe, if not resolved.

I have a client who was on four mood stabilizers and an antipsychotic when she first came in. When I did her labs, she had no Free T3, no testosterone, and she had no B_{12}. I remember thinking I don't know how she's here; I don't know how she's forming sentences; I don't know how she gets out of bed in the morning. Her labs were the worst I have ever, ever seen. She'd gone to therapy for years, but nothing was working. How could it?

We got her labs balanced, and now we've got her down to one antidepressant and one antipsychotic at the lowest therapeutic doses.

She tells me all the time, "I feel so much better. Things work."

Maybe it's because I'm the daughter of an engineer who's also a pilot, but I like to fix things. I have naturally gravitated towards areas in healthcare that are measurable, that are objective. Psychological conditions are measurable by survey, but many of them are subjective. I don't have a test for depression, I have an index.

I have found that what I'm measuring and what I'm correcting are independent risk factors for depression, in and of themselves. Low Vitamin D, low testosterone, dysfunctional thyroid either primary or secondary—these are measurable things that, when they go wrong, cause symptoms of depression.

During menopause and perimenopause, women will often fill out the boxes on the screenings that indicate they have depression in some form or fashion. That is one of the reasons why women aged 45 to 55 are described an antidepressant. But is it that she's not making enough neurotransmitters? Or is it that she has all these other things going wrong?

The index can't tell the difference. The index just says these are the symptoms.

Six months into my practice, I met a husband and wife. She'd had three kids and had suffered horrible postpartum depression with each one. When she came in, she'd gained 70 pounds and had what's called a pannus, where the belly folds over and can cover down to the mid-thigh.

Her labs were as bad as I expected, and I had a bad feeling she was suicidal, even though she denied suicidal ideation.

I talked to her husband who agreed with my assessment.

"We need to have a safety plan while I get her better," I said, going to explain that her energy would come back before her mood improved. That is the scariest time for someone who's suicidal, because now they've got enough wherewithal to do it, and they don't trust that they're going to ever get better.

We agreed that he would keep a close eye on her during the stages of improving her health. For six weeks, he never left her alone until he saw her mood visibly improve.

As we proceeded through the treatment process, I told him, I've got all kinds of different ways to do body composition and medical weight loss, but that hormonal pannus is a permanent change and to set some money aside because she was going to want her body back, and it would involve a tummy tuck.

That was two years ago.

She got her tummy tuck, and she wore a bikini this summer!

When you've had a decade of feeling off, your brain feels foggy, and the machine will move, but it's like turning these rusty wheels, and it just hurts; of course you're experiencing depression. I find over and over again that when people come to me on a couple of antidepressants or a mood stabilizer, as I treat them they often don't need it anymore. They made plenty of serotonin and norepinephrine and dopamine, but they didn't have what they needed in the rest of the body.

Depending on what's happened in your life, you might still need some therapy, but now it's in a body that's working. You're sleeping, you can actually have an orgasm, and you don't feel so tired you can't even get the grocery shopping done. If there's something you're working on, like better coping mechanisms, your marriage, better relationships with your kids, there is space to breathe in, to work in and be successful in, because all the noise of all the physical problems isn't taking up all of the space in the day.

HOW TO FIND A GOOD PRACTITIONER CHECKLIST

Biote® Pellets
- Biote® provider—providers must go through their training program, which includes a lengthy certification process.
- Established practice

Visit BioteMedical.com for a list of local providers by zip code.

General Women's Health—OB/GYN
- Highly recommended by friends, family, and in your community
- They have good credentials and experience
- They accept your insurance
- You feel comfortable with them
- They are knowledgeable about and open to bioidentical hormone therapy
- They're affiliated with a hospital you trust

Surgical and Non-Surgical Rejuvenation Providers:

- Look for labiaplasty, vaginoplasty, vaginal reconstruction, and vaginal rejuvenation before and after photos on a prospective surgeon's website.
- Is the doctor or someone in the practice trained and experienced in the specific procedure you want?
- Have they provided specific, individual pages on their website displaying their knowledge of the procedure? Can they provide proof of their expertise?
- Check patient reviews.
- Do they offer bioidentical hormone treatments?
- Do they offer Morpheus-V® and other nonsurgical vaginal rejuvenation options?
- Look for surgeons who are certified with the ABMS, and an additional cosmetic surgery board like the ABCS or ASPS. You should also look for a surgeon certified by the American Board of Obstetrics and Gynecology (ABOG).
- Make an appointment with at least two different surgeons.
- Note how you are treated by the office personnel. Do they treat you with respect, ask the right questions, explain, and help?
- Is the doctor easy to communicate with? Does he or she fully understand your feelings, what you are looking to accomplish both functionally and aesthetically? Do they discuss your anatomy specifically, reasonable expectations, recovery, anesthesia, etc.?
- Has your surgeon candidly discussed risk and given you careful and complete Informed Consent?
- Finances are important, and individual surgeon's fees can range, sometimes with experience.

Urology:
- Ask your primary care practitioner for a referral.
- Consider referrals and reviews of urologists in your area.
- Look for a urologist who supports bioidentical HRT.
- Check the urologist's website for education and specific specialties.
- Check insurance coverage.

Pelvic Floor Physical Therapy:
- Ask your health professional, a friend, or Google.
- Check out the clinic's website. The clinic website should put in the effort to answer common questions, explain what to expect at your first visit, educate you on what they do and how they can help, highlight the therapists' experience and credentials, and convey that their practice is a safe space.
- Reach out to the clinic, and they should connect you with one of the therapists for more detailed information.
- Find out if your insurance provider will cover pelvic PT sessions.
- Talk to and try more than one therapist. Personal comfort and fit are important.
- Find out if you'll get one-on-one attention. This is very intimate care. You shouldn't be left alone with exercises or a device while the therapist is off working on another patient or doing paperwork.

Psychology and Psychiatry
- Ask friends and family for referrals.
- Ask where he or she went to school. It doesn't matter where the therapist went, as long as it is an accredited school and not an online coaching certificate.
- What is her/her specialty? One therapist can't be all things to all people.
- Has he/she worked with people with your issues?
- What is their training? If he or she is trained, make sure it wasn't at a one-day seminar or a three-hour online course in psychoanalysis. If they call themselves an expert in a certain field, they need to be.
- Are they licensed? If so, I would still look up the license and make sure that it's in good standing.
- Ask if they are, or have ever been, in therapy. Do not get into therapy with someone who hasn't done their own work.
- Good therapists are not always convenient or cheap.
- Heed your intuition if it doesn't feel right. There are plenty of others out there.

TREATING ERECTILE DYSFUNCTION

Testosterone is the master hormone in charge of vascular health. Without testosterone, we see high blood pressure, cholesterol plaque formation, and a loss of vascular functionality—including in the erectile tissue.

Common wisdom is to pop a Viagra® before a sexual encounter, but without reestablishing underlying testosterone levels, men need a lot more ED medication, it doesn't work as well, and men have to keep increasing their dosage over time. Why? Because, again, you're trying to get blood to an area that needs testosterone for proper blood flow. Without testosterone, the blood vessels aren't going to have enough elasticity to either relax or contract. We need contraction outside of the penis, we need relaxation inside the penis, and we need contraction of the vessels at the exit of the penis, and that's how erectile blood flow works.

I treat a couple who got married later in life. They've been married now for eight or nine years, and they still look like newlyweds, always holding hands. Hers was a pretty easy, straightforward tune up. His, however, was a disaster: type 2 diabetes, on insulin, three blood pressure medications and a statin, because his cholesterol was terrible. He weighed 325 pounds, and he was supposed to weigh 190 pounds.

As I've said, kids bounce. People over 50 do not. Because he was in such a state, I set about getting him fixed up methodically and safely. When I put testosterone in a man, his blood pressure's going to normalize, but I don't know when. All of a sudden, that blood pressure's going to correct, and he's still going to be taking his blood pressure medicine. When it drops too low, then we have a problem. The same thing happens with diabetes—that blood sugar is going to correct. It's not going to get better in a linear fashion; the improvement happens in steps.

I always start very conservatively with clients who have multiple health challenges. We have a plan for blood pressure checks and blood sugar checks and tweak things as needed. It's taken two years, but he's down 85 pounds; he's off of his insulin; he's off one of his two oral diabetes medications; and he's only on Metformin (I really like Metformin for type 2 diabetes because it acts a little bit as a healthy anti-aging compound), a tiny bit of Lisinopril for his blood pressure, and no statin. He did carotid artery scans in the beginning, and he had some blockages, but they're completely gone. We were taught in school that as GFR, or glomerular filtration rate, falls, it never comes back. He's up 20 points, which is unheard of in a diabetic with kidney disease.

Oh, and he doesn't need his Viagra® anymore . . .

He and his bride report that their sexy time is much steamier.

In my practice, the first step is always to fix the testosterone. When that's still not quite enough, we start exploring additional remedies for erectile dysfunction.

VIAGRA® AND CIALIS®

Viagra® and Cialis® were developed as blood pressure medications. Researchers discovered the medication had a secondary effect of opening up the erectile vascular bed in the penis, which helped with erectile functionality. In other words, these drugs provided pressure in the pipes for a nice, solid erection. The erectile dysfunction medication frenzy took off from there.

I prescribe Cialis® over Viagra® for men who are receiving testosterone hormone replacement therapy because Viagra® plus testosterone can cause a postcoital (the time window just after orgasm/sex) drop in blood pressure. In other words, you have a great time in bed, then stand up, take two steps, and pass out.

It's not so sexy when you have to call 911 after sex!

One of my clients was on max-dose beta blockers because he'd had four vessels bypassed in his heart. He still needed Cialis® to have a really successful encounter. After treatment, he and his wife went on vacation, and he forgot his Cialis®. He was in the Caribbean where they only had Viagra®, which he couldn't take because it would drop his pressure too much.

Still, they were able to have sex over the weekend in the Caribbean, while using alcohol, which diminishes performance with no ED medication at all.

Z-WAVE™/SONIC WAVE DEVICE THERAPY

Pulse wave therapy was originally known as the GAINSWave. This modality of care utilizes sonic wave therapy to reduce inflammation and improve blood flow and has been used extensively by athletes. Major League pitchers will have sonic wave therapy on their throwing arm right after a game to reduce inflammation. It is used for plantar fasciitis, tendonitis, acute and chronic strains. You'll find these devices in the locker rooms of every professional sports team.

Over time, pulse wave therapy developed into a mainstay of erectile dysfunction therapy.

We use what is called Z-Wave™ pulse therapy for erectile dysfunction. The Z-Wave™ improves blood flow, gets new blood vessels coming into the area (neogenesis), and breaks up any micro-occlusions. So, it's pushing out inflammation and vascular occlusions in the capillary beds. It brings immediate blood flow to the area for healing, but it also causes the body to go through something called neogenesis—actual new blood vessels in the area.

Unlike the original pulse wave devices, which featured a tiny projectile on a long handheld wand that concentrated a lot of force into a small area, the Z-Wave™ has a larger projectile which allows an effective pulse wave with less force. In other words, the Z-Wave™ doesn't hurt like the old machines. Because it's sonic wave therapy on the penis, it's very important to utilize a device that's not uncomfortable!

People talk about clogged arteries in their neck or their heart. Anywhere you have vasculature, you can get a clog. When discussing how the Z-Wave™ breaks up micro occlusions in the capillary beds of the penis, one client described it as, "You're going to get the junk out of my junk."

Really, it's just physics, pipes, and pressure. It takes six treatments within two weeks, and clients get a remarkable change in blood flow and erectile functionality. Men get up to 80% of the improvements in the first two weeks, and then they continue to improve over the next three months. I find that during the first treatment, men look at the ceiling and they're not making eye contact. They just don't know what to do. By the third or fourth treatment, I can't get the door closed without the pants already coming off. They're just so happy to have their erectile strength back.

During the two weeks of treatment, the man is assigned homework. He has to reach orgasm every single day by himself or with a partner. It is important to get blood flow to the area for this treatment to work optimally, so we try to get it done in two weeks because he's going to run out of things to think about, and his partner is going to chase him off!

When the Z-Wave™ treatment is utilized after we've started hormone replacement therapy, it's typically curative. I don't have to repeat it. We're going on six years with a number of men, and they haven't needed a tune-up.

PUDENDAL NERVE DYSFUNCTION

Very rarely, men suffer from what is known as pudendal nerve dysfunction. The pudendal nerve comes off of the lowest part of the spinal column, called the cauda equina or horse tail. It's the lower lumbar and sacral area where you don't really have a spinal column anymore, it just sort of fans out in all these nerves. There are a variety of different back injuries where you can get what's called a tethered cord or compression. The pudendal nerve comes from the back to the front and feeds innervation of the pelvic floor, and specifically plays a huge role in erectile functionality.

It's pretty straightforward to screen for pudendal nerve dysfunction. When a man has an erection that disappears if he lays flat on his back, it may be indicative of this disorder. These men will typically masturbate on their side or standing up. It's really challenging for them to masturbate flat on their back because the erection is not just weaker, it's gone.

Some men with pudendal nerve dysfunction are out there chasing every solution. They order Viagra®, they use suction cups to try and pull blood into the penis. They try Z-Wave™ treatments and P shots—every procedure in the book. They go to a lot of time and expense, but they haven't seen a neurologist and/or urologist who specializes in pudendal nerve dysfunction.

Because the problem is actually in the back, not in the penis, I always want to make sure we rule it out. I ask very specific questions. *What's your favorite masturbatory position?* is not a question you expect to have to answer when you go in for your hormone check, but good screening is important for good outcomes.

I won't do a Z-Wave™ treatment or prescribe Cialis® for a man who has pudendal nerve dysfunction because it won't work. I send him on for further evaluation because he might need the back surgeon because of the tethered cord, or he might need a urological surgeon because the issue is further down.

ARTEROSIL®

I put men who have the Z-Wave™ treatment on a supplement called Arterosil®, which can stabilize vascular plaque within six weeks and eliminate it within six months. I treat high cholesterol and high blood pressure with Arterosil®. I treat Raynaud's (which is where the fingers and toes and nose go white and get cold) with it, and I also treat any form of erectile dysfunction with it.

We used to think blood vessels were a smooth pipe, but there's actually a layer deep on the inside which is the slime, or the slip, or the goo, and that's called the glycocalyx.

The glycocalyx, which is the middle of your blood vessels, should be eight nanometers thick. After you eat, you typically lose four nanometers no matter what. With age, the slippery, slimy layer starts to erode from eating too much sugar, smoking, drinking, and stress, which is highly inflammatory to the entire vasculature.

When you're a kid, your glycocalyx comes back within an hour. When you're an adult, it takes eight to ten hours, which is why intermittent fasting is so good for people with heart disease. When you don't have that glycocalyx, your cholesterol can stick whether or not it's high. So, it doesn't matter so much as the total cholesterol, as whether or not it can stick. Sticky cholesterol contributes to erectile dysfunction (penis and clitoris), carotid artery occlusions, etc.

Arterosil® is an over-the-counter supplement made by a compounding pharmacy in Florida that owns the U.S. patent. In other countries, it's available by prescription and has shown powerful improvement in the vasculature, including improving erectile dysfunction in the penis and the clitoris.

IT'S ALL GOOD

Testosterone is the master hormone in charge of vascular health in men.

I had a 69-year-old male client who came in having had a stent placed in his heart, which reoccluded 40% within the first year.

I did all of the things that I normally do, fixed his testosterone, which had fallen into the 300s. I fixed his Vitamin D and his thyroid, and he lost 20 pounds. I also started him on Arterosil® knowing that supplement would help keep his arteries clear and work to reduce any existing plaque.

Five years into his hormone journey with me, he had to have spinal stenosis surgery. Again, I can't fix everything, but everything goes better once I've fixed the things that I can fix. The anesthesiologist was terrified that his heart was full of clogs, and he wasn't going to survive the surgery, so they made him go get a heart catheterization to check.

He was completely clear.

Needless to say, it shocked the hell out of his cardiologist!

He's still doing great, and he still tells me about his sexy time, and he does this little stir the soup dance with it.

I know all is good.

John: Age 50

I started doing hormone replacement therapy five years ago. It was a game changer for me, but I was suffering sexual performance effects of chronic low testosterone and I needed something more to fix my erectile dysfunction.

Three years ago, I did six rounds of Z-Wave™ therapy over two weeks. It was very simple and easy to do. There were a couple instances where it got a little hot and we had to stop the treatment for 30 seconds to a minute, but overall the treatment is painless. By any stretch of the imagination there's no pain at all in it other than the feeling of having a hot pad in your groin.

As I said, I'd had erectile issues for years, and noticed a difference immediately after the first treatment as far as getting a full erection and better sex. As each treatment went along it got better and better. I would notice changes in stamina, length, and girth. By treatment four and five the changes in blood flow were very noticeable.

I'm really glad I went through the Z-Wave™ treatment. There's no harm in trying to get blood flow back to the organ that helps satisfy your sexual cravings.

SEXY TIME

Seven years ago, a couple came in to see me. They were former elite gymnasts who had become aerialists with Cirque du Soleil. They were in residence in one of the big shows in Las Vegas but often came to Denver to see family and wanted to see if I could help them. They had a couple of kids and loved performing but just couldn't seem to stay ahead of the injuries and were afraid they might have to retire.

I did their labs and all the things that I normally do and realized if I could get their testosterone back up, they probably could stay in their sport for at least another five years, maybe even ten. They were really excited about the possibility and got their pellets at the same time.

I got done and gave them my warning about not exercising, soaking, and no flexing the glutes for three to seven days.

"Well, what about our trapeze?" one of them asked.

"I don't know how you train for Cirque du Soleil, but I'll wager whatever you're doing involves your butt muscle," I said.

"No, the trapeze in our bedroom," said the other.

"Your what now?" I asked.

They proceeded to explain that they had a whole system set up in their bedroom with rings, chains, and bars. They were so excited about it and having so much fun with it, I almost felt bad making them wait a week to get back to their suburban bliss.

When I got home from work that evening and told my six-foot-five husband about my day, complete with trapeze, he said, "Oh my God, we have to get one."

"First of all, you're six-five, 220 pounds, you're going to rip it out of the ceiling, and then we're going to explain to some ER doctor why we need to be in traction from the trapeze in our bedroom," I said. "And, second, we are not acrobats."

We laughed ourselves silly, thinking about the two of us role playing in such an unlikely scenario, but with true admiration for the couple.

In truth, they were already set up for great success for HRT. Not only would the therapy extend their ability to perform in their careers, they already had the sexy time "infrastructure" set up at home.

PRIORITIZING INTIMACY

There's an old joke about relationships and marriage:

When you first get together you have anywhere sex. You get married and you have household sex. Once you start having kids you have bedroom sex. After your third kid you have hallway sex where you pass each other in the hall and say, "F— you!"

Sex doesn't have to devolve that way, but for so many, that's just what happens.

You do what you prioritize and plan for. A big part of planning for, say, exercise is to sign up and pay for a class because then you're going to show up. Even if it's just $5, no one likes to be out money. If you actually put something on the calendar and plan for it, chances are you're going to do it. Otherwise, it'll roll into tomorrow, and tomorrow rolls into next week. If you want to have regular, fantastic sexy time, guess what? You put that on the calendar, too.

If you have kids around, or curious onlookers, I don't suggest writing SEXY TIME in big block letters, but think up a code word and write it in ink. That way, you have a set plan. People may say it's not spontaneous, and therefore less fun, but if it's not on the calendar, you'll go a month or two months and you and your partner haven't touched each other.

Set aside a day and a time where you know you have the opportunity to have a great encounter. It shouldn't be at 10:00 p.m., because we're all tired and getting older by the minute. Even though we have all of our hormones fixed, we still have to get some sleep!

When you know sexy time is on Friday, for example, that automatically starts putting the pieces in place. You won't find yourself saying, "I'm so sweaty gross, and I think I've been wearing the same clothes for four days. You want to do what . . . ?"

When you decide together when you're going to have sex and it goes on the calendar, it becomes a sacred, special event that you plan around instead of the leftover item at the end of the day. You're in a place where you're thinking ahead. You know it's on the schedule, so you can pick up a new toy or a new outfit for you or your partner—men can dress up, too! You have this anticipatory buildup which is really fun. Some women don't feel sexy or want to get naked unless they've shaved their legs, had a bikini wax, or had their hair done. If you know that you're going to have sexy time on Friday, then schedule your bikini wax for Thursday, or blow dry your hair and shave your legs on Wednesday so you're ready.

The most important thing is maintaining your connection with your partner. We want to make sure that intimacy is a part of what we always cherish and plan for and prioritize.

SEXY MUSIC

In 2017, German researchers conducted a series of studies looking at music, sensuality, heightened awareness, and sexual pleasure. Sensuality is the experience of touch and interpretation of touch, so they looked at how people experience touch while certain music is playing. It turns out that if you play sexy music or music that's specifically sexy to you, the sense of touch is heightened tenfold. Just running your finger up your own arm becomes way more stimulating with certain music playing. When people listen to music they perceive as sexy, all stimulus is increased and is more pleasurable.

If you don't already have a playlist, create one. When you're driving down the road and a song comes on that gets you a little hot and bothered, snap a picture of it with your smartphone. (Only if it's safe while you're driving, of course) and then use it to start or add to a playlist. This can even be a precursor to sexy time.

You can have a few different playlists—the more romantic one, the more adventurous one. While you're at it, make sure your partner develops a playlist of their own. You can mix the songs back and forth together or put it on random. It doesn't matter as long as each of you gets the heightened, sensual awareness from the music. The songs that overlap can make for a super sexy playlist!

HABITS AND TRADITIONS

Sex isn't a leftover but a key component to a healthy adult relationship.

To that end, one of my clients, who is also a good friend, and her husband have *sexy Sundays*. They get up, they have coffee, and they go right back to bed. I know not to call her on Sunday mornings because she's not going to answer her phone. If I have anything I need to talk to her about, it has to wait until afternoon.

I know another couple who enjoy *Get your Freak on Fridays* every Friday night.

One of the best ones I've heard was from a set of parents who have kids in school and work from home. They take a sexy lunch break together. Planning sexy time when you're both awake and alert and have no interruptions is ideal for intimacy.

As for bigger traditions, I love the story of the "Naughty Stocking from one of my clients.

> **Renee: Age 49**
>
> *You know, Christmas Eve tends to be about family. Christmas morning is about the kids. When the kids were little, it was all we could do to get them to sleep in until seven a.m., and then there was the frenzy of going through the presents. There's often a big Christmas day meal followed by football and the inevitable food coma. It's all done by like seven or eight p.m. and the kids pass out early.*
>
> *That's when it's naughty stocking time!*
>
> *My husband and I have a glass of wine together and it's time for bedroom gifts. It's different every year— a vibrator, a new toy, outfits, or a risqué card game. Some of the things in the naughty stocking end up in*

> *the regular rotation, and some definitely don't work out. It doesn't matter. The point is for us to enjoy alone time together. One of the great gifts of Christmas is the intimacy we share with each other.*

If you don't celebrate Christmas, this particular tradition is easily modified for Hanukkah, Valentine's Day, Summer Solstice—you name it. Pick it, name it, and then have it be a tradition.

FIELD TRIP

During my first live seminar after the COVID shut down, I found out that about half the room of women over 50 didn't own a toy or a vibrator.

"If I fix your hormones and you don't have a toy, you're going to get carpal tunnel," I warned them.

We all howled with laughter, especially as we piled into cars. The next thing I knew, I had 25 women on a field trip to the adult store. The manager took us around and taught us everything from the difference between a rumble and a trill to the various toys out there for her and for him.

Everyone went home with something new, and it was so much fun.

ADULT STORE

There are basically two ways to shop for a sexy time toys—in person or online.

Online, you pick from what the retailer offers and hope for the best. It's way more anonymous, but there's no checking out the merchandise and there are no returns (for obvious reasons).

ONLINE ADULT STORE OPTIONS

- Adameve.com
- Pyramidcollection.com
- Amazon.com

If you go to one of the bigger adult stores, you are basically walking into a superstore filled with every imaginable toy, costume, device, and accoutrement for adult pleasure. If you've never shopped for toys in person, you do need to know that they will open the box, take out the vibrator, put in the batteries or plug it in to the charger, and turn the device on to full go mode to make sure it works. If that's too embarrassing, you may want to order online, but I suggest you work up the courage to go in person, so you can see and feel what's there and get the products you think you'll like the best.

Take your partner, take your friends, have a good time.

TOY STORE

There are hundreds of different vibrators designed for female genitalia—big ones, little ones, pointy ones, round ones, and ones with extra parts. There's something called a Rabbit which gives internal and external stimulus at the same time. There are also dildos of various shapes, sizes, and colors. (A dildo doesn't have a vibratory component to it and is designed to be inserted to simulate intercourse.) You need to pay attention to size. Is it going to fit you? Are you small? Are you medium? You don't want something that's too small, that's just annoying. You don't want something too big, that's just painful. And shape really matters. Do you have a clitoris that's so sensitive to touch that you orgasm fast? If so, you're going to want more of a round tip. If you have a clitoris that maybe has atrophied a bit or you have a little nerve loss or maybe that's just the way you were born, you want a little more pointy model because then that's going to get you a much more targeted stimulus.

There are two different types of vibration that you can purchase. One is a trill, and one is a rumble. A trill is more high-pitched and a rumble is deep-pitched. A trill is a really fast vibration that's not very penetrating. A rumble has a slower, deeper vibratory response. Some vibrators come with both.

Within a trill and a rumble there are different settings. There's constant, there's ramping up, and ramping down. There are different modes and different intensities, like how loud or soft within the trill or the rumble it is.

And then does it need batteries? Does it have a rechargeable cord? Is it waterproof? Do you have a hot tub? Do you have a pool? Do you have a soaker tub? Some of the waterproof ones can be really fun.

Over time, you may need to switch over to more of a rounded tip if you're using it only on the glans clitoris (the protruding, sensitive part of the clitoris often called "the clit"). And then if it's an intravaginal vibrator, typically you want the end to lift up. The G-spot, which is the tail end of the clitoris where it meets the end of the vaginal vault, is usually not right at the end of the vibrator. If a woman were to palpate her own vaginal vault and were to hook up and in around the pubic bone, that's where the G-spot is. So, you want the vibrator to go in and up toward the woman's belly button. A straight vibrator is not as successful at getting the G-spot as one that sort of curves.

I recommend starting with vibrators that aren't really long and that stretch the vaginal opening and hit the G-spot or the tail of the clitoris. Depth is not as stimulating. Which is why for a man's penis to hit the G-spot, usually the woman is on all fours and it's posterior entry. Missionary style tends to not hit the G-spot but will hit the clitoris.

I say try them all out by putting them on the inside of your wrist or the top of your head. You have more nerve endings on your scalp than you do in your clitoris or your penis, so trying a vibrator out in your scalp is going to really give you an idea of the stimulus.

TOYS FOR MEN

There are anal vibrators, surrogate vaginas and a horseshoe shaped vibrator which goes around the base of the penis and tucks underneath the scrotum. The base of the penis continues below the scrotum and testicles and toward the anus where it becomes the perineum. That area isn't typically stimulated in a sexual encounter with a partner. The horseshoe gets that little bit of penile tissue closer to the anus, which can be very exciting. A lot of people use that during a sexual encounter, particularly during oral sex, so the man has his vibrator as well.

EDGING

Edging (also known as teasing, surfing, or peaking) is the practice of stopping yourself from reaching orgasm just before you "fall off the cliff" into sexual climax. Edging can be done once, twice, or multiple times during a sexual encounter.

This practice was first discussed as a tool for sexual health in a 1956 paper published in the *Journal of Sexual Medicine* by James H. Semans who introduced the "stop-start method" to help people last longer before reaching orgasm.

The practice is accomplished by stopping sexual stimulation just before orgasm, waiting about 30 seconds, and then reengaging with your partner or stimulating yourself again, repeating until you're ready to orgasm.

Edging can have benefits during sexual encounters with a partner or for improving masturbation particularly by learning more about yourself and what feels good through all the states of sexual response. In 1966, William Masters and Virginia Johnson proposed a four-stage model of human sexual response based on 10,000 participants including:

1. Excitement. The skin starts to flush, heart rate is elevated, muscles can tense and blood flow engorges the penis or clitoris and vagina.

2. Plateau. Everything that happened in the Excitement stage gets even more intense, and the feeling of orgasm is imminent. This is the time to be ready to stop or slow down stimulation when utilizing edging.

3. Orgasm. Orgasm is a series of nerve and muscle responses resulting in sexual climax, feelings of ecstasy, increased lubrication in the vagina, and ejaculation from the penis.

4. Resolution. After orgasm, tissues return to their non-aroused sizes and colors, and heart rate and respiratory rate return to normal. This also includes the refractory period—a temporary stretch of time where you can't get aroused again, typically a few hours to a day/days.

According to the International Society for Sexual Medicine, edging can increase the intensity of orgasm in some people. This can apply to sex with a partner or masturbation, and including a period of edging during sex could help build up excitement and make the climax more satisfying.

Successful edging occurs by changing or lowering intensity just before orgasm. This might include changing position, stopping stimulation entirely, or slowing down the pace of activity. Having longer sexual encounters can also shift the focus away from orgasm and change the dynamics towards connecting with your partner. This may allow people to spend longer enjoying the process of stimulation.

According to a 2014 study, females who masturbate are more likely to achieve orgasm during sex. Practicing edging during masturbatory efforts may make it easier to reach orgasm. Additionally, people who experience premature ejaculation may find edging beneficial because it can increase the duration of sex before orgasm.

Sex and talking about sexual preferences is sometimes difficult for couples. Edging and communicating preferences during edging can allow opportunities for people to try new activities, discover new ways of touching or stimulating each other, and provides opportunities for people to talk about their sexual interests and learn about each other.

SEXY MUSIC PLAYLISTS

Songs that make me feel sexy:

_____
_____
_____
_____
_____
_____
_____
_____

Songs that make my partner feel sexy:

_____
_____
_____
_____
_____
_____
_____
_____

ATTACHMENT

Another aspect of sexual wellness and satisfaction comes in the form of attachment, as in how you bond to and feel intimate with your partner. There are different types of attachment, definitions of those types, and many studies on attachment and how it affects your sexual encounters. For this book, I'm going to use secure versus insecure attachment styles with insecure attachment style further broken down into insecure anxious attachment and insecure avoidance attachment styles.

Attachment style theory proposes that the way adults experience romantic attachment actually is formed early on in childhood and modeled on early relationships with parents or caregivers.

Secure: People who have strong attachments in early childhood, usually in healthy, safe, loving environments, form secure (trusting) attachments and, as adults, tend to gravitate towards healthy, safe, loving romantic relationships.

Insecure Anxious: People who spend their early childhood years with inconsistent parenting, have periods of abandonment, or caregivers who are affectionate sometimes, but cold and distant other times often form insecure (mistrust based) anxious attachment styles. As a result of the fear of abandonment, insecure-anxious-attachment people often want to merge completely with their partner, which can interfere with intimacy as the partner will crave space.

Insecure Avoidance: People raised with one extreme form of care or the other as in completely smothering caregivers or completely emotionally avoidant or absent caregivers often grow up to be emotionally avoidant. They have an underlying fear of rejection, which can make them "closed off" from their own inner emotional state and often struggle with expressing their feelings.

Research consistently shows that people with insecure attachment styles (anxious or avoidance) score lower on sexual satisfaction surveys, and it is helpful to know why these attachment styles get in the way of great sex. Through questionnaires, people with insecure anxious attachment styles experience a higher number of intrusive negative thoughts during encounters, distracting them away from erotic stimulus and their own bodily sensations. Additionally, people with insecure avoidance attachment style may even dislike sexual activity altogether as they can find the dependence on their partner to achieve sexual satisfaction a trigger to their own feelings of estrangement or alienation.

Basically, great sex happens when you get out of your head and into your body. A critical piece of sexual satisfaction is in the mindfulness of the encounter: staying in the "here and now." Securely attached people enter a sexual encounter from a place of trust and safety, allowing for both partners to be fully present and attuned to their own body and that of their partner.

Studies show that therapy or coaching can help distressed couples reach satisfying and healthy sexual relationships by both addressing attachment-insecurity issues as well as strengthening the relationship and creating more positive emotional experiences in and out of the bedroom. That means, if you are struggling with attachment and sexual satisfaction, it is a great time to utilize a therapist or couples coach who specializes in sexual wellness. If therapy isn't available, practicing mindfulness in and out of the bedroom is a fantastic way to work toward staying in the moment with your partner and increasing sexual satisfaction.

An Interview with Nancy Hamilton:

Nancy is a relationship coach with over 35,000 hours of relationship coaching and teaching relationship skills to couples. She has been on the Dr. Phil Show, NBC Dateline and ABC Nightline. She co-authored a book called THE SUCCESS FORMULA with Jack Canfield and has multiple programs for couples coaching. Nancy holds a bachelor's degree in psychology and humanities from the University of Colorado, Boulder, and a master's degree in social work from Smith College in Massachusetts.

Nancy: *I was a therapist for 25 years and I've been a coach for almost ten. Therapy is about why you're the way you are. Coaching is about what you are going to do about it. I bring everything I learned as a therapist into my coaching practice, so people kind of get the best of both worlds.*

Kimberly: *I love that you focus on solutions.*

Nancy: *People want to know how they can get better quickly, which is why I developed my brand, called* Better by Tonight.

Kimberly: *Tell me about* Better by Tonight.

Nancy: *Better by Tonight is based on the idea that there are skills you can learn right away that will have an immediate impact on your relationship. I work with people on managing complex change. You have to have a vision for that change, you have to have skills, incentives, resources and an action plan.*

When it comes to relationships you need to know what your vision is for an improved relationship, you need to write it as if it's already happening in present tense. For instance: we have fabulous sex *even if you're not having fabulous sex right now. I teach couples communication skills and conflict management skills, how to be more engaged and responsive to each other, and how to increase their self-awareness. I help couples redefine what their incentives are. Hopefully we get to a place where they want to help each other be or become the best versions of themselves.*

What you do, Kimberly, is a huge resource that I access and share with all of my clients. I can teach you all the best relationship skills in the world, but if you have wacky hormones or your partner isn't firing on all eight cylinders in terms of what's happening with them hormonally, then you're not going to have a good love life, you're not going to have a good sex life, and you're not going to have a good connection with your partner.

It really does start with biology.

Kimberly: *Can you talk a little bit about attachment and things you do for your clients in that realm?*

Nancy: *Attachment styles form in childhood between zero and two years old. It has to do with your caretakers and whether or not they consistently came when you cried, inconsistently came when you cried, or they were all over you.*

I'm a twin and our sister is 22 months older than we are, so my mom had three kids under the age of two. Sometimes my mom could get to me and sometimes she couldn't. That basically drove me towards more of an anxious attachment style in my love relationships as an adult. If my mom had just been all over me, like anticipating every need—it doesn't have to be your mom, but in my case it was my mom, my primary caregiver—I might have developed more of an avoidant attachment style as an adult.

If she came consistently when I cried —if, more often than not, she was able to meet my needs when I had them then, I would have become more of a securely attached adult. Which is just much more go with the flow, you don't really worry about your partner being absent, you don't have abandonment issues. A secure attachment style is something you find within a committed sexual relationship where both people had caregivers that came consistently when they needed them. The securely attached couples don't end up in therapy because things go pretty well. They're able to meet each other's needs and communicate what they need.

The problem is anxiously attached adults usually find avoidantly attached adults. Anxiously attached adults can be kind of clingy, they can fear abandonment. The primary question for an anxiously attached adult is are you there for me? Are you going to be there for me? And if you're not there physically then it means you're not there at all, and then they panic. *An anxiously attached person sometimes can use sex to get approval. And to reassure themselves that their partner desires them and that they're going to be okay. It's not the healthiest thing but it makes sense. If you didn't know if somebody was going to be there when you were a child it would make sense that you would be an intimate relationship where you don't know if the person's going to be there, because you're trying to get it right as an adult what you didn't get as a child.*

The avoidantly attached adult is somebody who, like I said earlier, was probably overwhelmed with attention. Not that you can have too much care, but the avoidantly attached person learned that intimacy can be overwhelming and smothering. And so the avoidantly attached adult spends a lot of time approaching and avoiding. This person might come on very strongly at the beginning of a relationship with a lot of love bonding and charisma and attention and time, but once they get into the intimate relationship, it's very overwhelming so then they start distancing behaviors. They don't want to snuggle after sex, they don't want to call if they're in a dating relationship. Avoidantly attached adults may engage in affairs because they don't have to dive deep into intimacy in an affair. They can engage in a lot of fantasy. Even when they're with their partner, an avoidantly attached person will employ a lot more fantasy so that they're not really getting attached emotionally with the person that they're with, they're fantasizing about somebody else. The other thing that avoidantly attached adults do is they use porn in an extensive way instead of just as an add-on to somebody's intimate life.

Like I said, the anxiously attached people and the avoidantly attached people tend to get together and those are the couples who wind up in my office because one person usually wants sex too much, one person doesn't want sex as much, they can't get that feeling of fulfillment and safety that the securely attached couple gets.

The good news about all of this is that it can change. If you happen to be with an anxiously attached adult and you happen to be with a securely attached adult, you become more securely attached. If you're in an anxiously and avoidantly attached relationship and you get coaching from the right person who understands these things, then you both can become more securely attached because you can negotiate and communicate. When things don't feel good you raise your hand and you say, "Hey, when it feels like you're being needy with me I just want to pull away. Can we talk about ways that you can feel safe and I can feel not smothered?"

Kimberly: How long do people usually spend in a coaching environment before they start seeing improvements in their sexy time?

Nancy: If we go back to the managing complex change model, the sooner that they learn the skills and can practice the skills and get support from me in using the skills the sooner they're going to see improvement. I had one couple that had been sexless for about a year and they came to see me. Their communication was a mess. They had a lot of conflict. I called them Mr. and Mrs. Bickerson. They were both really frustrated. Neither one of them was getting what they wanted and there wasn't anything happening in the bedroom.

Once we talked about their communication styles and I taught them some new skills, I really encouraged them to plot out time for each other. I'm a big proponent of date night. I think it was three or four sessions after our first session where we had been working on the relationship and the communication skills and they actually played strip poker on date night.

Kimberly: Fantastic.

Nancy: That's a big, gigantic step going from no sex to strip poker. They just felt like once they had the communication squared away, they felt more playful and they felt relieved and they felt like they could experiment. I think the humor of it kind of broke the ice because after you've been in a sexless period it's awkward. There needs to be some kind of icebreaker situation.

Kimberly: I love that.

Nancy: It happens pretty quickly using the managing complex change model because you're being very intentional about the process. Nobody wants to be in therapy or coaching forever, so usually people really like the Better by Tonight style.

Kimberly: *What else should people know about you or about your style of coaching or about your own journey?*

Nancy: As you know, I'm your number one biggest fan. About five years ago I was really trying to explore in my personal life how I could hit on all eight cylinders. I realized that biologically speaking I had never had my hormones checked. I'd had two children and I was perimenopausal. Actually, I was postmenopausal. I went to see you and it turned out that I had really, really low testosterone. It was a negative 2.5.

Kimberly: *I had actually never seen that before.*

Nancy: I know, that was totally nuts. It totally explained my sleeplessness, my low libido, the fact that I couldn't really gain a lot of muscle. And just my overall vitality, I just kind of felt dead. Not to be too dramatic about it, but I just kind of felt like I was in survival mode. Once I started treatment with you I just kind of woke up. I feel and have felt kind of like a teenage girl ever since. I love the benefits that I'm having in my own sex life. I feel a lot of desire, I feel a lot of satisfaction. It's just a wonderful feeling with that. I also love that it protects me against Alzheimer's and cardiovascular disease, and both of those things run in my family.

When I recommend that couples go see you it's because I've experienced all these wonderful things myself. And, like I said earlier, I can teach them all these great skills but if they are not right hormonally it's not going to do any good.

Kimberly: *You've got to start with the building blocks before you build. It's like trying to build a house without a foundation. It's not going to stand.*

Nancy: You do. You actually do. I'm all about hormones. I teach them that intimacy is all about safety. And how we go about getting that safety can sometimes be dysfunctional. As in anxious and avoidant and attached styles. But the goal is the same, the goal is safety.

Also, it has to be said, the cell phone is really the mistress of the 2000s. It's very addictive, as we all know. It's really hard to put it away. But that's something that I really encourage people to do, is to have kind of a screen free zone. I think the shared meals together is a perfect time to do that. I go out to dinner and I see these couples that are on their cell phones and they're not paying any attention to each other, and it just makes me really sad. I want to give them my business card.

Kimberly: *Because they're going to need you.*

Nancy: *They are, they're going to need me. Well, yeah, then they wonder where did our relationship—where did the wheels come off the wagon? I can say, well, it was when you guys couldn't put your phones down.*

Kimberly: *This is all fantastic. Thank you so much.*

Nancy: *You're welcome, and I'm thrilled to be a part of this project. I think this book has needed to be written for a long time. I love that you're bringing in the attachment styles. The couple that was playing strip poker after a few sessions with me nicknamed me the fairy godmother of F-ing.*

Kimberly: *Oh, God, I love that.*

Nancy: *My job is not to keep couples together, my job is to help teach them skills and to help them make a conscious decision of what they want to do in their relationship. I think great sex is the glue to any good relationship, any great relationship.*

LET'S DO IT!

As the saying goes, "Necessity is the mother of all invention." When I started down the path to hormone health, my needs were very basic: I needed my hormones optimized just so I could get out of the wheelchair. I needed to get better so I could be a part of my own life again instead of just surviving. But then I got better and better and realized that so many men and women needed the very same thing, so I started Cunningham Clinic and completely changed my approach to healthcare.

In sharing my knowledge about hormone health and how to live in a body that actually works, it became abundantly clear that people and healthcare providers weren't talking about how to live in a body that can have great sex. Humans are, for the most part, pack animals. We crave connection and great sex is a big part of that connection.

It's time to talk to your partner about what works for you. It's time to talk to a certified bioidentical hormone replacement therapy healthcare provider about what isn't working for you. Get your labs drawn and start with fixing the biology. Then, talk about what you can do to regain functionality and fun. This book is a jumping off point to start or continue the conversation about sexual wellness and satisfaction because *Great Sex Never Gets Old!*

FREQUENTLY ASKED QUESTIONS

Q: I've just moved into town and I've been on pellets for years. I just need more.

A: If you come in with a copy of your chart or you fill out a release of records information, I fax it over to your prior practice, and they fax me records, we can keep you on schedule for your next round of pellets. Fair warning though, I never assume that anybody else is as nerdy as I am about this though, so I always check labs again to make sure everything is exactly where it should be.

Q: Do you take insurance?

A: No. I'm a full-fledged health care practice. I just don't take insurance or do primary care anymore.

Q: What happens if I stop doing my hormones?

A: If you are a woman and you stop taking your hormones, you will go through the symptoms of hormone withdrawal. That is the definition of menopause. If you are a man and you stop taking your hormones, you will go through similar symptoms including fatigue, worsening pain, loss of muscle and sexual dysfunction. In other words, you'll age fairly quickly.

Q: If I fix my hormones will it completely fix my sleep?

A: Fixing sleep is a multifaceted process. A lot of times, we have to put clients on the cortisol reset plan, which is a combination of no caffeine after 10:00 a.m., including chocolate, no alcohol, no energy drinks at all, exercising six out of seven mornings a week for at least 45 minutes for women. Men can do it in 20 minutes. And then the only thing in the afternoons and evening would be like yin yoga because for what we're trying to do, cortisol peaks in the morning. Getting sleep is kind of like playing the piano. You can't just sit down and play. You've got to practice. So, there's something called good sleep hygiene that many people don't practice. They're drinking coffee until 5:00 p.m., or they're doing those power drink shots in the afternoon just so they can get to that unattainable finish line.

So, the long answer is that, yes, fixing hormones will start you on your way to better sleep but we may well need a few more interventions to get your sleep "fixed".

Q: How long will it take for me to feel "all better"?
A: Some people feel a difference as early as three weeks in, and some start to feel a difference in a few months. Either way, you'll likely continue to improve and feel better over the first two years of receiving HRT before stabilizing at a new, improved baseline health.

Q: What will it cost me on average to do pellet therapy the first year? Subsequent years?
A: Pellets are around $385 for women, three times a year and around $565-$750 for men, three times a year or less. Some clients need pellets more often and may come in as much as four times per year. Additionally, there are labs throughout the year including the $300 annual panel and then periodic follow up labs that run $125-$200.

Q: How young is too young to start HRT? How old?
A: I recommend starting to check an annual blood panel around age 35 but can check younger if someone is symptomatic of low

hormones. There is not a "too old" for HRT, and testosterone's contributions to muscle tone, balance, strength, and wellness are vital to healthy, independent aging. My oldest patient is currently 87 years old, and I fully intend to be someone's oldest patient one day as I'm never going without my hormones.

Q: What should I expect from my primary care doctor in terms of knowledge and appreciation for this path of HRT?
A: That depends on whether or not your primary care provider has read and/or researched bioidentical HRT and pellet therapy. I partner with many providers who support their patients' paths to wellness.

Q: My (male) partner needs help, but he's being stubborn about coming in. Any suggestions?
A: Have him just get the labs and then compare his results to the range in this book, rather than comparing them to the "reference range" on the lab printout.

Q: What is the best way to coordinate your care for my autoimmune condition with that of my other providers?
A: We always work with other providers to make sure that specific conditions are treated via a team approach. Just sign the release of information between the two practices, and we can coordinate care between providers.

Q: How do I know for sure if I'm in perimenopause or menopause?
A: The lab called FSH (follicle stimulating hormone) is a good indicator. If the FSH is above 40, that's usually menopause. Menopause

is often defined as an FSH above 40 and the absence of a menstrual cycle for at least 12 months. For women taking oral birth control pills, we would need to stop that medication for two to four weeks, then draw the blood to see if she is perimenopausal or menopausal.

Q: Will this cure the inability to have an orgasm?
A: Maybe. If the person was able to have an orgasm prior to perimenopause and/or menopause, and there has not been any trauma to the area associated with the anorgasmia, then it is possible that improving hormones will return the body to a state where orgasm is possible.

Q: Does testosterone help men with premature ejaculation as well as erectile function?
A: Absolutely though those measures can take up to a year to see the full improvements when starting HRT. Men who experience premature ejaculation can benefit from practicing edging once their testosterone has been optimized, and men who experience erectile dysfunction may need Z-Wave™ or other therapies to regain function once their testosterone has been optimized.

Q: Do you have any specific recommendations for same sex couples?
A: Not specifically—the gender of a person's partner doesn't change the goals for optimizing hormones and functionality. The goal is always to help the person live in a body that functions.

Q: I don't live in Denver or near Cunningham Clinic, how do I find a provider who is certified in bioidentical hormone replacement therapy?

A: To find a provider near you that is also Biote® certified, go to www.biotemedical.com and search on "Find a Provider" by your zip code. That will generate a list of providers close to your home that you can then meet to see which one is the best fit for you.

Q: Can I be treated at Cunningham Clinic if I don't live in Colorado?
A: Yes. We have many clients who choose to fly or drive to Denver three times a year for pellet therapy. It is simple enough to get labs in their hometown via a remote draw through LabCorp, but it really is most convenient for the client if they have a healthcare provider close to home.

REFERENCES

Abraham, G.E. "Facts about iodine and autoimmune thyroiditis." *The Original Internist* 15, no. 2 (2008): 75–76.

Adair, F., and J. Herrmann. "The use of testosterone propionate in the treatment of advanced carcinoma of the breast." *Annals of Surgery* 123 (1946): 1023–35.

Agoff, S., P. Swanson, H. Linden, S. Hawes, and T. Lawton. "Androgen receptor expression in estrogen receptor-negative breast cancer." *American Journal of Clinical Pathology* 120 (2003): 725–31.

Agrawal, A., M. Jelen, Z. Grzelenek, et al. "Androgen Receptor as a prognostic and predictive factor in breast cancer." Folia Histochemica et Cytobiologica 46 (2008): 269–276.

Aliano, Steven. "Women's Pain: Taking a Closer Look at the Disparity." *Practical Pain Management* (August 14, 2018).

Ambler, D. R., E. J. Bieber, and M. P. Diamond. "Sexual function in elderly women: a review of current literature." *Reviews in Obstetrics Gynecology* 5, no. 1 (2012): 16–27.

REFERENCES

Ando, S., F. De Amicis, V. Rago, A. Carpino, M. Maggiolini, M. Panno, and M. Lanzino. "Breast cancer from estrogen to androgen receptor." *Molecular and Cellular Endocrinology* 19 (2002): 121–128. Breastcancer.org.

Aspinall, Mara G., and Richard G. Hamermesh. "Realizing the Promise of Personalized Medicine." *Harvard Business Review* (October 2007).

Avenell A, Mak JC, O'Connell D. "Vitamin D and vitamin D analogues for preventing fractures in postmenopausal women and older men." Cochrane Database Syst Rev. 2014 Apr 14;2014(4).

Beaulieu, N., Brassard, A., Peloquin, K., et.al. Why do you have sex and does it make you feel better? Integrating attachment theory, sexual motives, and sexual well-being in long-term couples. *Journal of Social and Personal Relationships.* Vol 39, 12, 2022.

Bell, James R., Kimberley M. Mellor, Amanda C. Wollermann, Wendy T. K. Ip, Melissa E. Reichelt, Sarah J. Meachem, Evan R. Simpson, and Lea M. D. Delbridge. "Aromatase Deficiency Confers Paradoxical Postischemic Cardioprotection." *Endocrinology* 152, no. 12 (December 1, 2011): 4937–4947

Bianchi, V. E. "The Anti-Inflammatory Effects of Testosterone," *Journal of the Endocrine Society* 3, no. 1 (October 22, 2018): 91–107.

Biondi, B. "The normal TSH reference range: What has changed in the last decade?" *Journal of Clinical Endocrinology & Metabolism* 98, no. 9 (2013): 3584–3587.

Booth SL, Centi A, Smith SR, Gundberg C. "The role of osteocalcin in human glucose metabolism: marker or mediator?" *Nat Rev Endocrinol.* 2013 Jan;9(1):43-55.

Brincat M, et al. "The role of vitamin D in osteoporosis." *Maturitas.* 2015 Mar;80(3):329-32.

Burt LA, et al.,. "Effect of High-Dose Vitamin D Supplementation on Volumetric Bone Density and Bone Strength: A Randomized Clinical Trial." *JAMA.* 2019 Aug 27;322(8):736-745.

Carruthers, M., T.R. Trinick, and M.J. Wheeler. "The validity of androgen assays." *Aging Male* 10 (2007):165-72. Elliott, Ivo, Mayfong Mayxay, Sengchanh Yeuichaixong,

Cerillo, A., S. Bevilacqua, S. Storti, M. Mariani, E. Kallushi, A. Ripoli, et al. "Free triiodothyronine: a novel predictor of postoperative atrial fibrillation." *European Journal of Cardiothoracic Surgery* 24, no. 4 (2003): 487–492.

Chardes, T., N. Chapal, D. Bresson, C. Bes, V. Giudicelli, M. P. Lefranc, et al. "The human anti-thyroidperoxidase autoantibody repertoire in Graves' and Hashimoto's autoimmune thyroid diseases." *Immunogenetics* 54 (2002): 141–57.

REFERENCES

Cheang, M., S. Chia, D. Voduc, D. Gao, S. Leung, J. Snider, et al. "Ki67 index, HER2 status, and prognosis in clients with luminal B breast cancer." *Journal of the National Cancer Institute* 101 (2009): 736–750.

Chlebowski, R.T., Anderson, G. L., Aragaki, A.K., Manson, J. E., Stefanick, M. L., Pan, K., Barrington, W., Kuller, L. H. , Simon M. S., Lane, D., Johnson, K. C., Rohan, T. E., Gass, M.L.S., Cauley, J. A., Paskett, E.D., Sattari, M., Prentice, R.L. "Association of Menopausal Hormone Therapy With Breast Cancer Incidence and Mortality During Long-term Follow-up of the Women's Health Initiative Randomized Clinical Trials". *JAMA.* 2020 Jul 28; 324(4): 369–380.

Chlebowski. R.T., Kuller, L.H., Prentice, R.L., Stefanick, M.L., Manson, J.E., Gass, M., Aragaki, A.K., Ockene, J.K., Lane, D.S., Sarto, G.E., Rajkovic, A., Schenken, R., et al., for the WHI Investigators. "Breast Cancer after Use of Estrogen plus Progestin in Postmenopausal Women." *N Engl J Med.* 2009 Feb 5;360(6):573-87.

Choi, J., S. Kang, S. Lee, and Y. Bae. "Androgen receptor expression predicts decrease survival in early stage TNBC." *Annals of Surgical Oncology* 22, no. 1 (2015): 82–89.

Collins, L., K. Cole, J. Marotti, R. Hu, S. Schnitt, and R. Tamimi. "Androgen receptor in breast cancer in relation to the molecular phenotype." *Modern Pathology* 24 (2011): 924–931.

Collins, P. "Effects of testosterone on Coronary Vasomotor Regulation." *Circulation* 100 (1999): 1690–1696.

Coluzzi, F., D. Billeci, M. Maggi, and G. Corona. "Testosterone deficiency in non-cancer opioid-treated clients." *Journal of Endocrinological Investigation* 41, no. 12 (2018): 1377–1388.

Cooper, A., and B. B. Cooper. A treatise on dislocations, and on fractures of the joints. London: Churchill, 1822. Davison, S. "Androgens in Women." *Journal of Steroid Biochemistry & Molecular Biology* 85 (2003): 363–366.

Cranenburg EC, et al. "The circulating inactive form of matrix Gla Protein (ucMGP) as a biomarker for cardiovascular calcification." *J Vasc Res*. 2008;45(5):427-36.

Danzi, S., and I. Klein. "Potential uses of T3 in the treatment of human disease." *Clinical Cornerstone* 7, supplement 2 (2005): S9–15.

Dart, D. A., J. Waxman, E. O. Aboagye, and C. L. Bevan. "Visualising androgen receptor activity in male and female mice." *PLOS One* 8, no. 8 (August 7, 2013).

Davis, Susan R. "Is testosterone important for women as they age?" *Maturitas* 100 (2017): 95.

Davison, S. L., R. Bell, S. Donath, J. G. Montalto, and S. R. Davis. "Androgen levels in adult females: changes with age, menopause, and oophorectomy." *Journal of Clinical Endocrinology & Metabolism* 90 (2005): 3847–3850.

REFERENCES

Dimitrakakis, C., D. Zava, S. Marinopoulous, A. Tsigginou, A. Antsaklis, and R. Glaser. "Low salivary testosterone levels in clients with breast cancer." *BMC Cancer* 10 (2010): 547.

Dimitrakakis, C., R. Glaser, and A. York. "Beneficial effects of testosterone therapy in women measured by the validated Menopause Rating Scale (MRS)." *Maturitas* 68, no. 4 (2011): 355–361.

Dimitrakakis, C., R. Jones, A. Liu, and C. Bondy. "Breast cancer incidence in postmenopausal women using testosterone in addition to usual hormone therapy." *Menopause* 11 (2004): 531–535.

Donovitz GS. "Low complication rates of testosterone and estradiol implants for androgen and estrogen replacement therapy in over 1 million procedures." *Ther Adv Endocrinol Metab.* 2021 May 27; 12: 1-11.

Donovitz, Gary, MD, et al. "Testosterone Insufficiency and Treatment in Women: International Expert Consensus."

Donovitz, G., Cotton, M. "Breast Cancer Incidence Reduction in Women Treated with Subcutaneous Testosterone: Testoterone Therapy and Breast Cancer Incidence Study." *Eur J Breast Health.* 2021 Mar 31;17(2):150-156.

Dunn, Donna, PhD, CNM, FNP-BC (assistant professor), and Carla Turner, DNP, ACNP-BC (instructor). "Hypothyroidism in Women." *Nursing For Women's Health*, vol. 20 (2016): 93-96.

El Hadidy, E. M., et al. "Impact of severity, duration and etiology of hyperthyroidism on bone turnover markers and bone mineral density in men." *BMC Endocrine Disorders* 11 (2011): 2–7.

Elhomsy, G., and E. Staros, eds. "Antithyroid Antibody." *Laboratory Medicine* (2014).

Endocrine Society. "Testosterone improves verbal learning and memory in postmenopausal women." *ScienceDaily* (June 17, 2013).

Escobar-Morreale, H. F., et al. "Replacement therapy for hypothyroidism with thyroxine alone does not ensure euthyroidism in all tissues, as studied in thyroidectomized rats." *Journal of Clinical Investigation* 96, no. 6 (1995): 2828–38.

Escobar-Morreale, H. F., F. E. del Rey, M. J. Obregon, and G. M. de Escobar. "Only the combined treatment with thyroxine and triiodothyronine ensures euthyroidism in all tissues of the thyroidectomized rat." *Endocrinology* 137, no. 6 (1996): 2490–2502.

Feldman, Henry A., Christopher Longcope, Carol A. Derby, Catherine B. Johannes, Andre B. Araujo, Andrea D. Coviello, William J. Bremner, and John B. McKinlay. "Age Trends in the Level of Serum Testosterone and Other Hormones in Middle-Aged Men: Longitudinal Results from the Massachusetts Male Aging Study." *Journal of Clinical Endocrinology & Metabolism* 87, no. 2 (February 1, 2002): 589–598.

REFERENCES

Finkle, W. D., S. Greenland, G. K. Ridgeway, et al. "Increased risk of non-fatal myocardial infarction following testosterone therapy prescription in men." *PLOS One* 9, no. 1 (January 29, 2014).

Florencio-Silva, Rinaldo, Gisela Rodrigues da Silva Sasso, Estela Sasso-Cerri, Manuel Jesus Simões, and Paulo Sérgio Cerri. "Biology of Bone Tissue: Structure, Function, and Factors That Influence Bone Cells." *BioMed Research International* 2015, no. 421746 (2015).

Forman, L. J., V. Tingle, S. Estilow, and J. Cater. "The response to analgesia testing is affected by gonadal steroids in the rat." *Life Science* 45, no. 5 (1989): 447–454.

Fraser, W. D., D. Biggart, St. J. O'Reilly, H. W. Gray, J. H. McKillop, and J. A. Thompson. "Are biochemical tests of thyroid function of any value in monitoring clients receiving thyroxine therapy?" *British Medical Journal* 293 (1986): 1373.

Friedman E. The New Testosterone Treatment. Buffalo: Prometheus Books, 2013. Glaser, R. "Reduced breast cancer incidence in women treated with subcutaneous testosterone." *Maturitas* 76 (2013): 342–349.

Friedman, E. *How You and Your Doctor Can Fight Breast Cancer, Prostate Cancer, and Alzheimer's.* New York: Prometheus, 2013.

Garin, M. C. "Subclinical thyroid dysfunction and hip fracture and bone mineral density in older adults: The cardiovascular health study." *Journal of Clinical Endocrinology & Metabolism* 99, no. 8 (2014): 2657–64.

Gibbons, J.B., Norton, E.C., McCullough, J.S., Meltzer, D.O., Lavigne, J., Fielder, V.C., Gibbons, R.D. "Association between vitamin D supplementation and COVID-19 infection and mortality." *Scientific Reports* volume 12, Article number: 19397 (2022).

Gibson, Carolyn J., PhD, MPH, Yongmei Li, PhD, Daniel Bertenthal, MPH, Alison J. Huang, MD, MAS, and Karen H. Seal, MD, MPH. "Menopause symptoms and chronic pain in a national sample of midlife women veterans." *Menopause* 26, no. 7 (July 2019): 708–713.

Glaser, R. "Testosterone therapy in women: Myths and misconceptions." *Maturitas* 74, no. 3 (2013): 230–34.

Glaser, R. L., A. E. York, and C. Dimitrakakis. "Abstract P6-13-02: Reduced incidence of breast cancer with testosterone implant therapy: A 10-year cohort study." *Cancer Research* 79, supplement 4 (February 15, 2019): P6-13-02.

Glaser, R. L., C. Dimitrakakis, and A. G. Messenger. "Improvement in scalp hair growth in androgen-deficient women treated with testosterone: a questionnaire study." *British Journal of Dermatology* 166, no. 2 (2012): 274–278.

Glaser, R., et al. "Testosterone implants in women: Pharmacologic doses for a physiologic effect." *Maturitas* 74, no. 3 (2013): 179–184.

Glaser, Rebecca, and Constantine Dimitrakakis. "Rapid response of breast cancer to neoadjuvant intramammary testosterone-anastrozole therapy: neoadjuvant hormone therapy in breast cancer." *Menopause* (June 1, 2014).

Glaser, Rebecca, et al. "Testosterone therapy in women: Myths and misconceptions." *Maturitas* 74, no. 3: 230–234.

Goldstein, Irwin, et al. "Hypoactive Sexual Desire Disorder." *Mayo Clinic Proceedings* 92, no. 1 (2017): 114–128.

Gorres, G., et al. "Bone mineral density in clients receiving suppressive doses of thyroxine for differentiated thyroid carcinoma." *European Journal of Nuclear Medicine* 23, no. 6 (1996): 690–692.

Gouras G. K., H. Xu, R. S. Gross, et al. "Testosterone reduces neuronal secretion of Alzheimer's beta-amyloid peptides." Proceedings of the National Academy of Sciences of the United States of America 97, no. 3 (2009): 1202–1205.

Greenblatt RB, Suran RR. "Indications for hormonal pellets in the therapy of endocrine and gynecic disorders." *Am J Obstet Gyncol.* 1949; 57:249-301.

Heiman, J. R., Long, J. S., Smith, S. N., Fisher, W. A., Sand, M. S., & Rosen, R. C. (2011). Sexual satisfaction and relationship happiness in midlife and older couples in five countries. *Archives of Sexual Behavior*, 40(4), 741–75.

Henderson, B. "Hormonal Carcinogenesis," *Carcinogenesis* 21, no. 3 (2000): 427–433.

Hennemann, R. D., E. Friesema, et al. "Plasma membrane transport of thyroid hormones and its role in thyroid hormone metabolism and bioavailability." *Endocrine Reviews* 22, no. 4 (2001): 451–476.

Herrmann, J., and F. Adair. "The effects of testosterone propionate on carcinoma of the female breast with soft tissue metastasis." *Journal of Clinical Endocrinology & Metabolism* 6 (1946): 769–775.

Hilborn, E. "Androgen receptor expression predicts beneficial tamoxifen response." *British Journal of Cancer* 114 (2016): 248–255.

Hoang, T. D., C. H. Olsen, V. Q. Mai, P. W. Clyde, and M. K. Shakir. "Desiccated thyroid extract compared with levothyroxine in the treatment of hypothyroidism: A randomized, double-blind, crossover study." *Journal of Clinical Endocrinology & Metabolism* 98, no. 5 (2013): 1982–90.

Hofling, M., A. Hirschberg, L. Skoog, et al. "Testosterone inhibits estrogen/progestogen-induced breast cell proliferation in postmenopausal women." *Menopause* 14 (2007): 183.

Holick MF. "Vitamin D deficiency." *N Engl J Med.* 2007 Jul 19;357(3):266-81.

Hossein-Nezhad A, Holick MF. "Vitamin D for health: a global perspective". *Mayo Clin Proc.* 2013 Jul;88(7):720-55.

REFERENCES

Howlader, N., A. Noone, M. Krapcho, D. Miller, K. Bishop, C. Kosary, et al. "SEER Cancer Statistics Review, 1975–2014." https://seer.cancer.gov/csr/1975_2014, based on November 2016 SEER data submission.

Islam, R. M., R. J. Bell, S. Green, and S. R. Davis. "Effects of testosterone therapy for women: a systematic review and meta-analysis protocol." *Systematic Reviews* 8, no. 1 (January 11, 2019).

Jameson, J., A. Fauci, D. Kasper, S. Hauser, D. Longo, and J. Loscalzo, eds. *Harrison's Principles of Internal Medicine*, 20th edition. New York: McGraw Hill, 2018.

Jones, T. Hugh, et al. "The effects of testosterone on risk factors for, and the mediators of, the atherosclerotic process." *Atherosclerosis* 207, no. 2, (2009): 318–327.

Jonklaas, J., Bianco, A.C., Bauer, A.J., Burman, K.D., Cappola, A.R., Celi, F.S., Cooper, D.S., Kim, B.W., Peeters, R.P., Rosenthal, M.S., Sawka, A.M. Guidelines for the Treatment of Hypothyroidism: Prepared by the American Thyroid Association Task Force on Thyroid Hormone Replacement. *Thyroid.* 2014 Dec 1; 24(12): 1670-1751.

Jude, E.B., Ling, S.F., Allcock, R., Yeap, B.X.Y., Pappachan, J.M. "Vitamin D Deficiency Is Associated With Higher Hospitalization Risk From COVID-19: A Retrospective Case-control Study." *J Clin Endocrinol Metab.* 2021 Oct 21;106(11).

Jung-Ho, P., et al. BMJ Open 7, no. 11 (2017). Koelling, Sebastian, and Nicolai Miosge. "Sex Differences of Chondrogenic Progenitor Cells in Late Stages of Osteoarthritis." *Arthritis & Rheumatism* 62, no. 4 (January 13, 2010): 1077-87.

Kharrazian, D. *Why Do I Still Have Thyroid Symptoms When My Lab Tests Are Normal: A Revolutionary Breakthrough In Understanding Hashimoto's Disease And Hypothyroidism.* New York: Morgan James Publishing, 2010.

Khaw, Kay-Tee, Mitch Dowsett, Elizabeth Folkerd, Sheila Bingam, Nicholas Wareham, Robert Lafortune D, Girard M, Bolduc R, Boislard MA, Godbout N. Insecure Attachment and Sexual Satisfaction: A Path Analysis Model Integrating Sexual Mindfulness, Sexual Anxiety, and Sexual Self-Esteem. *J Sex Marital Ther.* 2021. Kim, H. K., S. Y. Kang, Y. J. Chung, J. H. Kim, and M. R. Kim. "The Recent Review of the Genitourinary Syndrome of Menopause." *Journal of Menopausal Medicine* 21, no. 2 (2015): 65–71.

Krotkiewski, M. "Thyroid hormones and treatment of obesity." *International Journal of Obesity* 24 (2000): S116–S119.

Kuchenbaecker, K., J. Hopper, D. Barnes, et al. "Risks of breast, ovarian, and contralateral breast cancer for BRCA1 and BRCA2 mutation carriers." *Journal of the American Medical Association* 317, no. 23 (2017): 2402–2416.

REFERENCES

LaRosa, John C. "Lipids and cardiovascular disease: Do the findings and therapy apply equally to men and women?" *Women's Health Issues* 2, no. 2: 102–113.

Larsen, P. R. "Thyroid-pituitary interaction: feedback regulation of thyrotropin secretion by thyroid hormones." *New England Journal of Medicine* 306, no. 1 (1982): 23–32.

LeBoff MS, et al. "Supplemental Vitamin D and Incident Fractures in Midlife and Older Adults." *N Engl J Med.* 2022 Jul 28;387(4):299-309.

Lehmann, B., J. Bauer, J. Schafer, C. Pendleton, L. Tang, K. Johnson, et al. "PIK3CA mutations in androgen receptor positive triple negative breast cancer confers sensitivity to the combination of PI3K and androgen receptor inhibitors." *Breast Cancer Research* (2014).

Levkovich, I., A. Gewirtz-Meydan, K. Karkabi, and L. Ayalon. "When sex meets age: Family physicians' perspectives about sexual dysfunction among older men and women: A qualitative study from Israel." *European Journal of General Practice* 25, no. 2 (2019): 85–90.

Leylan-Jones, B. "Human Epidermal growth factor receptor 2 positive breast cancers and CNS metastasis." *Journal of Clinical Oncology* 27 (2009): 5278–86.

Lim, V. S., C. Passo, Y. Murata, E. Ferrari, et al. "Reduced triiodothyronine content in liver but not pituitary of the uremic rat model: demonstration of changes compatible with thyroid hormone deficiency in liver only." *Endocrinology* 114, no. 1 (1984): 280–286.

Lovejoy, J. C., F. A. Bray, M. O. Bourgeois, R. Macchiavelli, J. C. Rood, C. Greesen, and C. Partington. "Exogenous androgens influence body composition and regional body fat distribution in obese post-menopausal women—a clinical research center study." *Journal of Clinical Endocrinology & Metabolism* 81 (1996): 2198–2203.

Luben, Ailsa Welch, and Nicholas Day. "Endogenous Testosterone and Mortality Due to All Causes, Cardiovascular Disease, and Cancer in Men, European Prospective Investigation into Cancer in Norfolk (EPIC-Norfolk) Prospective Population Study." *Circulation* 116 (November 26, 2007): 2694–2701.

Luidens, M., S. Mousa, F. Davis, H. Lin, and P. Davis. "Thyroid hormone and angiogenesis." *Vascular Pharmacology* 52, no. 3-4 (2010): 142–145.

Maclaren, K., et al. "The safety of post-menopausal testosterone therapy." *Women's Health* (2012): 263–275.

Maia, A. L., et al. "Pituitary cells respond to thyroid hormone by discrete, gene-specific pathways." *Endocrinology* 136 (1995): 1488–94.

Manolagas, S. C., C. A. O'Brien, and M. Almeida. "The role of estrogen and androgen receptors in bone health and disease." *Nature Reviews Endocrinology* 9, no. 12 (2013): 699–712.

REFERENCES

Matthews, K. A., S. L. Crawford, C. U. Chae, et al. "Are changes in cardiovascular disease risk factors in midlife women due to chronological aging or to the menopausal transition?" *Journal of the American College of Cardiology* 54, no. 25 (2009): 2366–2373.

Mazziotti, G., L. D. Premawardhana, A. Parkes, H. Adams, P. Smyth, D. Smith, W. Kaluarachi, et al. "Evolution of thyroid autoimmunity during iodine prophylaxis—the Sri Lankan experience." *European Journal of Endocrinology* 149 (2003): 103–110.

McNamara, K. M., T. Yoda, Y. Miki, N. Chanplakorn, S. Wongwaisayawan, P. Incharoen, et al. "Androgen pathway in triple negative invasive ductal tumors." *Cancer Science* 104 (2013): 639–646.

McNichols, N.K. "How Attachment Style Impacts Sexual Satisfaction." Psychology Today. Posted December 23, 2021.

Mearini, L., A. Zucchi, et al. "Prevalence of low testosterone (total testosterone less than 300 ng/dl) is as high as 38.7% in males over 45 in out-client primary care populations." *World Journal of Urology* 31, no. 2 (November 9, 2011): 247–252.

Meeker, John D., and Kelly K. Ferguson. "Urinary Phthalate Metabolites Are Associated with Decreased Serum Testosterone in Men, Women, and Children from NHANES 2011–2012." *Journal of Clinical Endocrinology & Metabolism* (2014): 2014–2555.

Mensah-Nyagan, A. G., L. Meyer, V. Schaeffer, C. Kibaly, and C. Patte-Mensah. "Evidence for a key role of steroids in the modulation of pain." *Psychoneuroendocrinology* 34, supplement 1 (2009): S169–S177.

Metcalfe, K., S. Gershman, P. Ghadirian, H. Lynch, C. Snyder, N. Tung, et al. "Contralateral mastectomy and survival after breast cancer in carriers of BRCA1 and BRCA2 mutations: retrospective analysis." *British Medical Journal* (2014): 348.

Morgentaler, Abraham, et al. "Fundamental Concepts Regarding Testosterone Deficiency and Treatment." *Mayo Clinic Proceedings* 91, no. 7 (2016): 881–896.

Mulligan, T., M. F. Frick, Q. C. Zuraw, A. Stemhagen, and C. McWhirter. "Prevalence of hypogonadism in males aged at least 45 years: the HIM study." *International Journal of Clinical Practice* 60, no. 7 (2006): 762–769.

Mitchell, A.L., Hegedus, L., Zarkovic, M., Hickey, J.L., Perros, P. Patient satisfaction and quality of life in hypothyroidism: An on-line survey by the British thyroid foundation. *Clin Endocrinol* (Oxf). 2021 Mar; 94 (3): 513-520.

Naessen, Tord, Ulrika Sjogren, Jonas Bergquist, Marita Larsson, Lars Lind, and Mark M. Kushnir. "Endogenous Steroids Measured by High-Specificity Liquid Chromatography-Tandem Mass Spectrometry and Prevalent Cardiovascular Disease in 70-Year-Old Men and Women." *Journal of Clinical Endocrinology & Metabolism* 95, no. 4 (April 1, 2010): 1889–97.

Nappi, Rossella E., et al. "The CLOSER (Clarifying Vaginal Atrophy's Impact On Sex and Relationships) Survey: Implications of Vaginal Discomfort in Postmenopausal Women and in Male Partners." *The Journal of Sexual Medicine* 10, no. 9: 2232–41.

Nappi, R., Nijland, E.A. "Women's perception of sexuality around the menopause: Outcomes of a European telephone survey." *European Journal of Obstetrics and Gynecology and Reproductive Biology* 137, no. 1 ( ): 10–16. (2008).

Narayanan, R., and T. Dalton. "Androgen Receptor: A complex therapeutic target for breast cancer." *Cancers* 8 (2016): 108–125.

Nathanson, K. "Breast Cancer Genetics." *Natural Medicine* 7 (2015): 552–556.

Noh, S., J. Kim, and J. Koo. "Metabolic differences in estrogen receptor negative breast cancer is based on androgen receptor status." *Tumor Biol* 35 (2014): 8179–92.

North American Menopause Society. "Hormone Therapy Position Statement of the North American Menopause Society." *The Journal of the North American Menopause Society* 24, no. 7 (2017): 728–753.

Notelovitz, Morris. "Androgen effects on bone and muscle." *Fertility and Sterility* 77 (2002): 34–41.

Office of the Surgeon General. "Bone health and osteoporosis: A report of the Surgeon General." Rockville: US Department of Health and Human Services, 2004.

Onitilo, A., J. Engel, R. Greenlee, and B. Mukesh. "Breast cancer subtypes based on ER/PR and HER2 expression." *Clinical Medical Research* 7 (2009): 4–13.

Ortiga-Carvalho, T. M., et al. "Thyroid hormone receptors and resistance to thyroid hormone disorders." *National Review of Endocrinology* 10, no. 10 (2014): 582–591.

Papadimitriou, D. T. "The Big Vitamin D Mistake." *J Prev Med Public Health*. 2017 Jul; 50(4): 278–281.

Pastuszak, A. W. "Testosterone replacement therapy in clients with prostate cancer after radical prostatectomy." *Journal of Urology* 190 (2013): 639–644.

Pavlou, H., P. Kliridis, A. Panagiotopoulos, C. Goritsas, and P. Vassilakos. "Euthyroid sick syndrome in acute ischemic syndromes." *Angiology* 53, no. 6 (2002): 699–707.

Pepper, G. M., and P. Y. Casanova-Romero. "Conversion to Armour Thyroid from Levothyroxine improved client satisfaction in the treatment of hypothyroidism." *Journal of Endocrinology, Diabetes, and Obesity* 2, no. 3 (2014): 1055.

Pergola, C., A. Rogge, G. Dodt, H. Northoff, C. Weinigel, D. Barz, O. Radmark, L. Sautebin, and O. Werz. "Testosterone suppresses phospholipase D, causing sex differences in leukotriene biosynthesis in human monocytes." *The FASEB Journal* (2011).

Perou, C., T. Sorlie, M. Eisen, M. van de Rijn, S. Jeffrey, C. Rees, et. al. "Molecular portraits of human breast tumors." *Nature* 407 (2000): 748–752.

Persani, L. "Central Hypothyroidism: Pathogenic, diagnostic, and therapeutic challenges." *Journal of Clinical Endocrinology & Metabolism* 9, no. 7 (2012): 3068–78.

Peters, A., G. Buchanan, C. Ricciardelli, T. Bianco-Miotto, M. Centenera, J. Harris, et al. "Androgen receptor inhibits estrogen receptor-alpha activity and is prognostic in breast cancer." *Cancer Research* 69 (2009): 6131–40.

Peterson, S. J., A. Cappola, R. Castro, C. Dayan, A. Farwell, J. Hennessey, et al. "An Online Survey of Hypothyroid Clients Demonstrates Prominent Dissatisfaction." *Thyroid* (2018).

Qu, Q., Y. Mao, X. Fei, and K. Shen. "The impact of the androgen receptor expression on breast cancer survival." *PLOS One* 8 (2013): 1-8.

Quan, M. L. "Bone mineral density in well-differentiated thyroid cancer clients treated with suppressive thyroxine: A systematic overview of the literature." *Journal of Surgical Oncology* 79, no. 1 (2002): 62–70.

Raisz L.G. "Pathogenesis of Osteoporosis." *Journal of Clinical Investigation* 115, no. 12 (2005): 3318–25.

Rajendran, P., T. Rengarajan, J. Thangavel, et al. "The vascular endothelium and human diseases." *International Journal of Biological Sciences* 9, no. 10 (November 9, 2013): 1057–69.

Santen, R., W. Uyue, and D. Heitan. "Modeling of the growth kinetics of occult breast tumors." *Cancer Epidemiology, Biomarkers and Prevention* 21, no. 7 (2012): 1038–48.

Saravanan, P., and C. M. Dayan. "Thyroid autoantibodies." *Endocrinology and Metabolism Clinics of North America* 30 (2001): 315–337.

Sarrel, P., et al. "The Mortality Toll of Estrogen Avoidance: An Analysis of Excess Deaths Among Hysterectomized Women Aged 50 to 59 Years." *American Journal of Public Health* (July 18, 2013): e1–e6.

Savvas, M., J. W. Studd, S. Norman, A. T. Leather, T. J. Garnett, and I. Fogelman. "Increase in bone mass after one year of percutaneous oestradiol and testosterone implants in post-menopausal women who have previously received long-term oral oestrogens." *BJOG: An International Journal of Obstetrics & Gynaecology* 99 (1992): 757–760.

Scavello, I., E. Maseroli, V. Di Stasi, and L. Vignozzi. "Sexual Health in Menopause." *Medicina* (Kaunas) 55, no. 9 (September 2, 2019): 559.

REFERENCES

Scheyer, O., A. Rahman, H. Hristov, et al. "Female Sex and Alzheimer's Risk: The Menopause Connection." *Journal of Prevention of Alzheimer's Disease* 5, no. 4 (2018): 225–230.

Sharma, R., O. A. Oni, K. Gupta, et al. "Normalization of Testosterone Levels after Testosterone Replacement Therapy Is Associated With Decreased Incidence of Atrial Fibrillation." *Journal of the American Heart Association* 6, no. 5 (May 9, 2017)

Sharma, Rishi, Olurinde A. Oni, Kamal Gupta, Guoqing Chen, Mukut Sharma, Buddhadeb Dawn, Ram Sharma, Deepak Parashara, Virginia J. Savin, John A. Ambrose, and Rajat S. Barua. "Normalization of testosterone level is associated with reduced incidence of myocardial infarction and mortality in men." *European Heart Journal* 36, no. 40 (October 21, 2015): 2706–15.

Sheppard, M. C. "Levothyroxine treatment and occurrence of fracture of the hip." *Archives of Internal Medicine* 162, no. 3 (2002): 338–343.

Sherwin, Barbara B., et al. "Differential symptom response to parenteral estrogen and/or androgen administration in the surgical menopause." *American Journal of Obstetrics & Gynecology* 151, no. 2 (1965): 153–160.

Shimoyama, Cardiology (1993). Starr, M., Hypothyroidism type 2: The epidemic. Irvine: New Voice Publication, 2011.

Shores, M. M., A. M. Matsumoto, K. L. Sloan, and D. R. Kivlahan. "Low Serum Testosterone and Mortality in Male Veterans." *Archives of Internal Medicine* 166, no. 15 (2006): 1660–65.

Shufelt, C. L., and G. D. Braunstein. "Testosterone and the breast." *Menopause International* 14, no. 3 (2008): 117–122.

Simon, James, Irwin Goldstein, Noel Kim, et al. "The role of androgens in the treatment of genitourinary syndrome of menopause (GSM): International Society for the Study of Women's Sexual Health (ISSWSH) expert consensus panel review." *Menopause* (July 1, 2018).

Slomski A. "Which Postmenopausal Women Should Use Testosterone for Low Sexual Desire?" *Journal of the American Medical Association.* (published online January 22, 2020).

Stanczyk FZ, Shoupe D, Nunez V, Macias-Gonzales P, Vijod MA, Lobo RA. "A randomized comparison of nonoral estradiol delivery in postmenopausal women." *Am J Obstet Gynecol.* 1988 Dec;159(6):1540-6.

Stoffel, E. C., C. M. Ulibarri, J. E. Folk, K. C. Rice, and R. M. Craft. "Gonadal hormone modulation of mu, kappa, and delta opioid antinociception in male and female rats." *Journal of Pain* 6, no. 4 (2005): 261–274.

Strich, D., G. Karavani, S. Edri, and D. Gillis. "TSH enhancement of FT4 to FT3 conversion is age dependent." *European Journal of Endocrinology* 175 (2016): 49–54.

Studd, J., et al. "The relationship between plasma estradiol and the increase in bone density in postmenopausal women after treatment with subcutaneous hormone implants." *American Journal of Obstetrics & Gynecology* 163, no. 5 (1990): 1474–79.

Tennant, Forest, MD, PhD. "Hormone Therapies: Newest Advance in Pain Care." *Practical Pain Management* 11, no. 4 (2011): 98-105.

Tenover, J. S. "Effects of testosterone supplementation in the aging male." *Journal of Clinical Endocrinology & Metabolism* 75, no. 4 (October 1, 1992): 1092–98.

Thom MH, Collins WP, Studd JW. "Hormonal profiles in postmenopausal women after therapy with subcutaneous implants." *Br J Obstet Gynaecol.* 1981 Apr;88(4):426-33.

Toloza, F.J.K., Suarez, N.R.E., El Kawkgi, O., Golembiewski, E.H. et. Al. Patient Experiences and Perceptions Associated with the Use of Desiccated Thyroid Extract. *Medicina* (Kaunas). 2020 Apr; 56(4): 161.

Traish, Abdulmaged M., Linda Vignozzi, James A. Simon, Irwin Goldstein, and Noel N. Kim. "Role of Androgens in Female Genitourinary Tissue Structure and Function: Implications in the Genitourinary Syndrome of Menopause." *Sexual Medicine Reviews* 6, no. 4 (2018): 558.

University of California–San Francisco. "Testosterone Aids Older Men's Brains, UCSF Study Says." *ScienceDaily* (April 16, 2002).

University of Gothenburg, "Keeping active in middle age may be tied to lower risk of dementia." *ScienceDaily* (February 25, 2019).

Van Den Eeden, S. K. "Thyroid hormone use and the risk of hip fracture in women >/=65 years: A case-control study." *Journal of Women's Health* (Larchmt) 12, no. 1 (2003): 27–31.

Vera-Badillo, F. E., A. Templeton, P. deGouveia, I. Diaz-Padilla, P. Bedard, M. Al-Mubarak, et al. "Androgen receptor expression and outcomes in early breast cancer." *Journal of the National Cancer Institute* (2014).

Van Lankveld, J.J.D.M., Dewitte, M., Verboon, P., vanHooren, S.A.H. Associations of Intimacy, Partner Responsiveness, and Attachment-Related Emotional Needs with Sexual Desire. Front. *Psychol.*, 21 June 2021.

Vigen, R., C. I. O'Donnell, A. E. Barón, et al. "Association of Testosterone Therapy with Mortality, Myocardial Infarction, and Stroke in Men with Low Testosterone Levels." *Journal of the American Medical Association* 310, no. 17 (2013): 1829–36.

Walsh-Childers, K., H. Edwards, and S. Grobmyer. "Covering women's greatest health fear: Breast cancer information in consumer magazines." *Health Communication* 26, no. 3 (2011): 1–12, 209—220.

REFERENCES

Wentz, I., and M. Nowosadzka. *Hashimoto's Thyroiditis: Lifestyle Interventions For Finding And Treating The Root Cause.* White River Junction: Wentz, LLC, 2013.

White, H., et al. "Treatment of Pain in Fibromyalgia Clients With Testosterone Gel: Pharmacokinetics and Clinical Response." *International Immunopharmacology* 27, no. 2 (2015): 249–56.

Wilson, C. M., and M. J. McPhaul. "A and B forms of the androgen receptor are expressed in a variety of human tissues." *Molecular and Cellular Endocrinology* 120 (1996): 51–57.

Yingheng, L., B. Sherer, A. Redetzke, and M. Gerdes. "Regulation of arteriolar density in adult myocardium during low thyroid conditions." *Vascular Pharmacology* 52, no. 3–4 (2010): 146–150.

Zhang, Y., and J. M. Jordan. "Epidemiology of osteoarthritis" (published correction appears in Clinics in Geriatric Medicine. 29, no. 2 (May 2013): ix). *Clinics in Geriatric Medicine* 26, no. 3 (2010): 355–369.

Zmuda, J. *American Journal of Cardiology* 77 (1996): 1244–47. Atherosclerosis 130 (1997): 199–202.

ABOUT THE AUTHOR

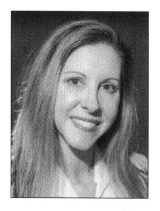

Kimberly Cunningham is a Board Certified Nurse Practitioner, providing healthcare in Colorado for over 20 years with a practice experience covering an array of settings including the emergency department, inpatient hospital care, skilled nursing facilities, internal medicine, and healthy aging clinics. She started Cunningham Clinic with a focus on integrating Western and European guidelines to help people look and feel better after suffering a life-changing injury that left her immobile for years. She started her own journey and recovery utilizing hormone replacement therapy, opened her own clinic, and now teaches other providers how to integrate hormone therapies into their own practices.

Cunningham Clinic offers both healthy aging solutions and aesthetic treatments. Highly skilled in procedures, Kimberly is often called on to provide injection services for complex patients and to teach other providers best practices and novel approaches when utilizing aesthetic treatments. Her passion for helping people to look and feel better is achieved through a conservative approach. Kimberly's goal is to help aesthetic clients achieve desired results with the minimum amount of intervention to achieve a natural correction and to avoid looking "done." First time clients can feel comfortable knowing she uses a "start low, go slow" approach and crafts clinic days to allow for longer visits and time to review each person's individual anatomy, age related changes and the best way to utilize aesthetic treatments to correct those changes.

EDUCATION

MS in Nursing: University of Colorado College of Nursing
BSN: University of Colorado College of Nursing
Biochemistry Focus: South Dakota School of Mines and Technology
Bachelor of Arts Degree in History: University of Florida

BOARD CERTIFICATION AND LICENSURE

American Academy of Nurse Practitioners: Board Certified Adult Nurse Practitioner
Advanced Practice Nurse: State of Colorado
Registered Nurse: State of Colorado

PROFESSIONAL AFFILIATIONS

University of Colorado, College of Nursing, Adjoint Faculty
Regis University, College of Nursing, Adjoint Faculty
Allergan Medical Institute (AMI), Trainer
Biote® Medical, Faculty
American Academy of Nurse Practitioners, Member
Colorado Nurses Association, Member
American Nurses Association, Member
Sigma Theta Tau Nursing Honorary, inducted 2004

HRT CHECKLIST FOR WOMEN AND MEN

Do I need to get my blood checked? If you check any of the below, it may be time to get a comprehensive set of labs.

<u>Women</u>
- ◊ Fatigue
- ◊ Mood swings/irritable
- ◊ Poor sleep
- ◊ Anxiety
- ◊ Joint pain or loss of muscle
- ◊ Loss of motivation or your "edge"
- ◊ Weight gain
- ◊ Low sex drive
- ◊ Night sweats
- ◊ Vaginal dryness
- ◊ Hot flashes
- ◊ Change in hair (loss, brittle, thinning)
- ◊ Worsening health or increased need for medications

Men

- ◊ Fatigue
- ◊ Mood swings/irritable
- ◊ Poor sleep
- ◊ Anxiety
- ◊ Joint pain or loss of muscle
- ◊ Loss of motivation or your "edge"
- ◊ Weight gain
- ◊ Low sex drive
- ◊ Loss or reduction of morning erections
- ◊ Change in hair (loss, brittle, thinning)
- ◊ Night sweats
- ◊ Worsening health or increased need for medications

Labs recommended for proper screening with some optimal levels/goals.

Women
- CBC
- Chemistry
- Vitamin D (Goal 70-100)
- Vitamin B_{12} (Goal 700-1000)
- TSH (Goal <2.0 and no symptoms)
- Free T3 (Goal 3.5-4.5)
- Free T4
- Total T4
- TPO Antibodies (thyroid antibodies) (Goal negative for Hashimoto's)
- Ferretin (Goal >40)
- Total testosterone (Goal 80-250 or 125-250 post pellet placement)
- Free testosterone (via LCMS/MS Assay) (Goal 7-15 pg/ml)
- FSH (follicle stimulating hormone)
- Estradiol
- Lipid panel (cholesterol)
- Hemoglobin A1C (Goal at or below 5.5)

Men
- ◊ CBC
- ◊ Chemistry
- ◊ Vitamin D (Goal 70-100)
- ◊ Vitamin B$_{12}$ (Goal 700-1000)
- ◊ TSH (Goal <2.0 and symptom free)
- ◊ Free T3 (Goal 3.5-4.5)
- ◊ Free T4
- ◊ Total T4
- ◊ TPO Antibodies (thyroid antibodies) (Goal negative for Hashimoto's)
- ◊ Total testosterone (Goal 900-1100 and elite athletes up to 1450 post pellet placement)
- ◊ Free testosterone (via LCMS/MS Assay) (Goal 150-200 pg/ml)
- ◊ Estradiol (Goal less than 50 and no symptoms of tearfulness or sore nipples)
- ◊ PSA (if over age 45) (Goal less than 3.0)
- ◊ Prolactin (Goal negative for prolactinoma risk)
- ◊ Lipid panel (cholesterol)
- ◊ Hemoglobin A1C (Goal at or below 5.5)

What happens after I start hormone replacement therapy?

<u>Women</u>
- ◊ More energy
- ◊ Improved focus and drive
- ◊ Better sleep
- ◊ Quicker recovery from workouts
- ◊ Muscle development from exercise
- ◊ Better sex drive
- ◊ Improved orgasms
- ◊ Vaginal tone
- ◊ Stronger pelvic floor
- ◊ Improved vaginal secretions
- ◊ Better bladder control
- ◊ Improved circulation
- ◊ Reduced risk of Alzheimer's, diabetes, cancer (including breast cancer), high blood pressure, coronary artery disease
- ◊ No more "olditis!"

Men

- ◊ More energy
- ◊ Focus and drive
- ◊ Better sleep
- ◊ Quicker recovery from workouts
- ◊ Muscle development from exercise
- ◊ Better sex drive
- ◊ Stronger erections
- ◊ Improved orgasms
- ◊ Stronger pelvic floor
- ◊ Improved circulation
- ◊ Reduced risk of Alzheimer's, diabetes, cancer, high blood pressure, coronary artery disease, prostate issues and erectile dysfunction
- ◊ No more "olditis!"

ACKNOWLEDGEMENTS

I will be forever grateful for the support of so many amazing people I have been fortunate to have in my life. Thank you to my friends and family who supported my practice, attended my lectures and even proofread all the versions of this book.

Special thanks to my husband, Steve, and our two kids, Abigail and Andrew, who carried more than their fair share these last months to allow me the time to complete this project. Steve you are my Superman, my soulmate and my home.

Like many providers, I would not be here without the education and guidance of my mentors, Doctors Bruce Dorr and David Watson, owners of Littleton Gynecology and Wellness in Littleton, Colorado. Both amazing physicians and humans, they spend countless hours as faculty members of Biote Medical providing training for bioidentical hormone replacement therapy as well as innovating new techniques to improve this modality of care.

Special thank you to Barbara Brooks, founder of Second Act Women. She is a champion of women 40, 50 plus, a force to be reconned with and the one who looked me straight in the eye and told me to write this book.

To my amazing team at Cunningham Clinic, I am beyond blessed to be surrounded by such a thoughtful, intelligent, dynamic and rock solid group. Together we have built a practice that is able to reach a large number of people and help them live healthier, stronger lives.

Finally, to the patients of Cunningham Clinic. Thank you for trusting us with your care and allowing us to walk alongside you along your own paths to wellness. Yours are the stories that fill these pages.